Diabetes
Information
for Teens

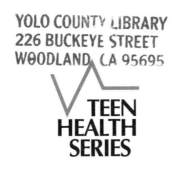

TEEN
HEALTH
SERIES

First Edition

Diabetes Information for Teens

Health Tips about Managing Diabetes and Preventing Related Complications

*Including Information about Insulin, Glucose
Control, Healthy Eating, Physical Activity, and
Learning to Live with Diabetes*

◆

Edited by Sandra Augustyn Lawton

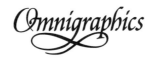

615 Griswold Street • Detroit, MI 48226

Bibliographic Note

Because this page cannot legibly accommodate all the copyright notices, the Bibliographic Note portion of the Preface constitutes an extension of the copyright notice.

Edited by Sandra Augustyn Lawton

Teen Health Series

Karen Bellenir, *Managing Editor*
David A. Cooke, M.D., *Medical Consultant*
Elizabeth Barbour, *Research and Permissions Coordinator*
Cherry Stockdale, *Permissions Assistant*
Dawn Matthews, *Verification Assistant*
Laura Pleva Nielsen, *Index Editor*
EdIndex, Services for Publishers, *Indexers*

* * *

Omnigraphics, Inc.

Matthew P. Barbour, *Senior Vice President*
Kay Gill, *Vice President—Directories*
Kevin Hayes, *Operations Manager*
Leif Gruenberg, *Development Manager*
David P. Bianco, *Marketing Director*

* * *

Peter E. Ruffner, *Publisher*

Frederick G. Ruffner, Jr., *Chairman*

Copyright © 2006 Omnigraphics, Inc.

ISBN 0-7808-0811-8

Library of Congress Cataloging-in-Publication Data

Diabetes information for teens : health tips about managing diabetes and preventing related
   complications including information about insulin, glucose control, healthy eating, physical
   activity, and learning to live with diabetes / edited by Sandra Augustyn Lawton.
      p. cm. -- (Teen health series)
   Summary: "Provides basic consumer health information for teens on diabetes, treatment
   methods, and coping strategies. Includes index, resource information and recommendations for
   further reading"--Provided by publisher.
   Includes bibliographical references and index.
   ISBN 0-7808-0811-8 (hardcover : alk. paper)
   1. Diabetes--Juvenile literature. 2. Diabetes in adolescence--Juvenile literature. 3. Diabetes
--Complications--Prevention--Juvenile literature.   I. Lawton, Sandra Augustyn. II. Series.
   RC660.5.D53 2006
   616.4'62--dc22
                                                                                            2005036597

The information in this publication was compiled from the sources cited and from other sources considered reliable. While every possible effort has been made to ensure reliability, the publisher will not assume liability for damages caused by inaccuracies in the data, and makes no warranty, express or implied, on the accuracy of the information contained herein.

This book is printed on acid-free paper meeting the ANSI Z39.48 Standard. The infinity symbol that appears above indicates that the paper in this book meets that standard.

Printed in the United States

Table of Contents

Part III: Diabetes And Related Health Concerns

Part IV: Day-To-Day Living With Diabetes

Part V: Coping With Feelings And Relationships

Part VI: If You Need More Information

Preface

About This Book

An estimated 18.2 million people in the United States—6.3 percent of the population—have diabetes. Of those, 13 million have been diagnosed and about 5.2 million are unaware of their condition. More than 200,000 people under 20 years of age have the disease. Uncontrolled or poorly controlled diabetes is associated with complications that can cause serious problems throughout the body, including nerve damage, loss of vision, amputation, kidney failure, and even death.

The teen years are especially important in the battle against diabetes. In adolescence, many young people with type 1 diabetes (also called juvenile diabetes or insulin-dependent diabetes) begin to take more personal responsibility for managing their condition. As they develop a better understanding of the disease process, they are better equipped to monitor and control blood sugar levels.

Teens also need to know about type 2 diabetes (non-insulin dependent diabetes). Although type 2 diabetes is traditionally associated with older people, recent statistics indicate that its prevalence among the young is increasing. Furthermore, the lifestyle choices teens make can have a direct impact on their risk of developing diabetes later in life.

Diabetes Information For Teens provides information about the different types of diabetes, risk factors, diagnostic procedures, and strategies used to manage the course of the disease, including the use of insulin and self-monitoring of blood glucose. It describes related health concerns and how to prevent complications. It offers practical tips about such topics as healthy eating, dining out, weight management, physical activity, sports participation, handling sickness or emergencies, and coping with feelings and relationships. For readers seeking more information, the book provides suggestions for further reading and a directory of diabetes resources.

How To Use This Book

This book is divided into parts and chapters. Parts focus on broad areas of interest; chapters are devoted to single topics within a part.

Part I: Basic Information About Diabetes begins with an overview and statistical facts about diabetes. It discusses the different types of diabetes and their risk factors, describes how various ethnic groups are affected, and concludes with a discussion about diabetes prevention.

Part II: Diabetes Treatment And Management reports on the tests and devices used to monitor diabetes and the medications most commonly used to control it. It explains the different roles of various health care providers, the use of glucose meters, insulin, and insulin delivery devices. Tips on site rotation for insulin injections and how to dispose of used insulin syringes and lancets are also included.

Part III: Diabetes And Related Health Concerns presents facts about some of the most common medical consequences of diabetes, including problems with the eyes, feet, skin, kidneys, nervous system, heart, and blood vessels. It also discusses hyperglycemia and hypoglycemia, conditions related to too much, or too, little blood sugar.

Part IV: Day-To-Day Living With Diabetes provides suggestions about healthy eating, weight management, physical activity, and other aspects of daily diabetes management that impact lifestyle. It addresses the special concerns of athletes with diabetes and discusses sports nutrition. Specific suggestions are also offered for dealing with diabetes away from home, either at school, at a job, at a restaurant, or while traveling.

Part V: Coping With Feelings And Relationships discusses the emotional challenges people with diabetes sometimes face, including depression, poor self-esteem, and difficulty in relationships with family and friends. A discussion regarding the benefits of self-advocacy is also included.

Part VI: If You Need More Information includes suggestions for additional reading and a directory of diabetes resources.

Bibliographic Note

This volume contains documents and excerpts from publications issued by the following government agencies: National Diabetes Education Program (NDEP); National Highway Traffic Safety Administration (NHTSA); National Institute of Diabetes and Digestive and Kidney Diseases (NIDDK); National Institute of Mental Health (NIMH); National Institutes of Health (NIH); National Library of Medicine; National Women's Health Information Center (NWHIC); Transportation Security Administration (TSA); U.S. Environmental Protection Agency (EPA); and the U.S. Food and Drug Administration (FDA).

In addition, this volume contains copyrighted documents and articles produced by the following organizations and publications: Allina Hospitals and Clinics; American Diabetes Association; Anorexia Nervosa and Related Eating Disorders; Australian Sports Commission; BD Consumer Healthcare; Canadian Diabetes Association; Children's Diabetes Foundation; Children's Diabetes Foundation of the North Bay; Children with Diabetes and Diabetes 123; Joslin Diabetes Center; Nemours Foundation; New Mexico State University Cooperative Extension Service; *Physician and Sportsmedicine*; R. A. Rapaport Publishing; Utah Department of Health—Tobacco Prevention and Control Program; and West Suffolk Hospitals NHS Trust.

Full citation information is provided on the first page of each chapter. Every effort has been made to secure all necessary rights to reprint the copyrighted material. If any omissions have been made, please contact Omnigraphics to make corrections for future editions.

Acknowledgements

In addition to the organizations listed above, special thanks are due to research and permissions coordinator Elizabeth Barbour and to managing editor Karen Bellenir.

About the *Teen Health Series*

At the request of librarians serving today's young adults, the *Teen Health Series* was developed as a specially focused set of volumes within Omnigraphics' *Health Reference Series*. Each volume deals comprehensively with a topic selected according to the needs and interests of people in middle school and high school.

Teens seeking preventive guidance, information about disease warning signs, medical statistics, and risk factors for health problems will find answers to their questions in the *Teen Health Series*. The *Series*, however, is not intended to serve as a tool for diagnosing illness, in prescribing treatments, or as a substitute for the physician/patient relationship. All people concerned about medical symptoms or the possibility of disease are encouraged to seek professional care from an appropriate health care provider.

If there is a topic you would like to see addressed in a future volume of the *Teen Health Series*, please write to:

Editor
Teen Health Series
Omnigraphics, Inc.
615 Griswold Street
Detroit, MI 48226

Locating Information within the *Teen Health Series*

The *Teen Health Series* contains a wealth of information about a wide variety of medical topics. As the *Series* continues to grow in size and scope, locating the precise information needed by a specific student may become more challenging. To address this concern, information about books within the *Teen Health Series* is included in *A Contents Guide to the Health Reference Series*. The *Contents Guide* presents an extensive list of more than 12,000 diseases, treatments, and other topics of general interest compiled from the Tables of Contents and major index headings from the books of the *Teen Health Series* and *Health Reference Series*. To access *A Contents Guide to the Health Reference Series*, visit www.healthreferenceseries.com.

Our Advisory Board

We would like to thank the following advisory board members for providing guidance to the development of this *Series*:

Dr. Lynda Baker, Associate Professor of Library and Information Science, Wayne State University, Detroit, MI

Nancy Bulgarelli, William Beaumont Hospital Library, Royal Oak, MI

Karen Imarisio, Bloomfield Township Public Library, Bloomfield Township, MI

Karen Morgan, Mardigian Library, University of Michigan-Dearborn, Dearborn, MI

Rosemary Orlando, St. Clair Shores Public Library, St. Clair Shores, MI

Medical Consultant

Medical consultation services are provided to the *Teen Health Series* editors by David A. Cooke, M.D. Dr. Cooke is a graduate of Brandeis University, and he received his M.D. degree from the University of Michigan. He completed residency training at the University of Wisconsin Hospital and Clinics. He is board-certified in internal medicine. Dr. Cooke currently works as part of the University of Michigan Health System and practices in Ann Arbor, MI. In his free time, he enjoys writing, science fiction, and spending time with his family.

Part One

Basic Information About Diabetes

Chapter 1

Diabetes Overview

Almost everyone knows someone who has diabetes. An estimated 18.2 million people in the United States—6.3 percent of the population—have diabetes, a serious, lifelong condition. Of those, 13 million have been diagnosed, and about 5.2 million people have not yet been diagnosed.

What is diabetes?

Diabetes is a disorder of metabolism—the way our bodies use digested food for growth and energy. Most of the food we eat is broken down into glucose, the form of sugar in the blood. Glucose is the main source of fuel for the body.

After digestion, glucose passes into the bloodstream, where it is used by cells for growth and energy. For glucose to get into cells, insulin must be present. Insulin is a hormone produced by the pancreas, a large gland behind the stomach.

When we eat, the pancreas automatically produces the right amount of insulin to move glucose from blood into our cells. In people with diabetes, however, the pancreas either produces little or no insulin, or the cells do not

About This Chapter: Excerpted from "Diabetes Overview," a publication of the National Diabetes Information Clearinghouse (NDIC), a service of the National Institute of Diabetes and Digestive and Kidney Diseases (NIDDK), National Institutes of Health (NIH), NIH Publication No. 05-3873, January 2005.

respond appropriately to the insulin that is produced. Glucose builds up in the blood, overflows into the urine, and passes out of the body. Thus, the body loses its main source of fuel even though the blood contains large amounts of glucose.

What are the types of diabetes?

These are the three main types of diabetes:

- type 1 diabetes
- type 2 diabetes
- gestational diabetes

Type 1 Diabetes: Type 1 diabetes is an autoimmune disease. An autoimmune disease results when the body's system for fighting infection (the immune system) turns against a part of the body. In diabetes, the immune system attacks the insulin-producing beta cells in the pancreas and destroys them. The pancreas then produces little or no insulin. A person who has type 1 diabetes must take insulin daily to live.

> **♣ It's A Fact!!**
> **Signs Of Diabetes**
>
> - Being very thirsty
> - Urinating often
> - Feeling very hungry or tired
> - Losing weight without trying
> - Having sores that heal slowly
> - Having dry, itchy skin
> - Losing the feeling in your feet or having tingling in your feet
> - Having blurry eyesight
>
> Source: Excerpted from "What Diabetes Is," a publication of the National Diabetes Information Clearinghouse (NDIC), a service of the National Institute of Diabetes and Digestive and Kidney Diseases (NIDDK), National Institutes of Health (NIH), February 2005.

At present, scientists do not know exactly what causes the body's immune system to attack the beta cells, but they believe that autoimmune, genetic, and environmental factors, possibly viruses, are involved. Type 1 diabetes accounts for about 5 to 10 percent of diagnosed diabetes in the United States. It develops most often in children and young adults, but can appear at any age.

Symptoms of type 1 diabetes usually develop over a short period, although beta cell destruction can begin years earlier. Symptoms include increased

thirst and urination, constant hunger, weight loss, blurred vision, and extreme fatigue. If not diagnosed and treated with insulin, a person with type
1 diabetes can lapse into a life-threatening diabetic coma, also known as
diabetic ketoacidosis.

Type 2 Diabetes: The most common form of diabetes is type 2 diabetes.
About 90 to 95 percent of people with diabetes have type 2. This form of
diabetes is associated with older age, obesity, family history of diabetes, previous history of gestational diabetes, physical inactivity, and ethnicity. About
80 percent of people with type 2 diabetes are overweight.

Type 2 diabetes is increasingly being diagnosed in children and adolescents.
However, nationally representative data on prevalence of type 2 diabetes in
youth are not available.

When type 2 diabetes is diagnosed, the pancreas is usually producing
enough insulin, but for unknown reasons, the body cannot use the insulin
effectively, a condition called insulin resistance. After several years, insulin
production decreases. The result is the same as for type 1 diabetes—glucose
builds up in the blood, and the body cannot make efficient use of its main
source of fuel.

The symptoms of type 2
diabetes develop gradually.
Their onset is not as
sudden as in type 1 dia-
betes. Symptoms may
include fatigue or
nausea, frequent
urination, unus-
ual thirst, weight
loss, blurred vision,
frequent infections,
and slow healing of
wounds or sores. Some
people have no symp-
toms.

♣ It's A Fact!!

About 206,000 young people under 20 years of age have diabetes. As
obesity rates in children continue to soar,
type 2 diabetes, a disease that used to be seen
primarily in adults over age 45, is becoming more
common in young people.

Source: Excerpted from "Resources on Children
and Adolescents," National Diabetes Education
Program, National Institutes of Health,
cited March 2005; available online at
http://www.ndep.nih.gov/diabetes/
youth/youth.htm.

Gestational Diabetes: Gestational diabetes develops only during pregnancy. Like type 2 diabetes, it occurs more often in African Americans, American Indians, Hispanic Americans, and among women with a family history of diabetes. Women who have had gestational diabetes have a 20 to 50 percent chance of developing type 2 diabetes within 5 to 10 years.

What are the tests for diagnosing diabetes?

The fasting plasma glucose test is the preferred test for diagnosing type 1 or type 2 diabetes. It is most reliable when done in the morning. However, a diagnosis of diabetes can be made after positive results on any one of three tests, with confirmation from a second positive test on a different day.

- A random (taken any time of day) plasma glucose value of 200 mg/dL or more, along with the presence of diabetes symptoms.

- A plasma glucose value of 126 mg/dL or more after a person has fasted for 8 hours.

♣ **It's A Fact!!**

To move away from basing the names of the two main types of diabetes on treatment or age at onset, an American Diabetes Association expert committee recommended in 1997 universal adoption of simplified terminology.

- Type 1 diabetes is the preferred name for:
  - Type I
  - Juvenile diabetes
  - Insulin-dependent diabetes mellitus
  - IDDM
- Type 2 diabetes is the preferred name for:
  - Type II
  - Adult-onset diabetes
  - Noninsulin-dependent diabetes mellitus
  - NIDDM

Source: Excerpted from "Diagnosis of Diabetes," a publication of the National Diabetes Information Clearinghouse (NDIC), a service of the National Institute of Diabetes and Digestive and Kidney Diseases (NIDDK), National Institutes of Health (NIH), NIH Publication No. 05-4642, January 2005.

- An oral glucose tolerance test (OGTT) plasma glucose value of 200 mg/dL or more in a blood sample taken 2 hours after a person has consumed a drink containing 75 grams of glucose dissolved in water. This test, taken in a laboratory or the doctor's office, measures plasma glucose at timed intervals over a 3-hour period.

Gestational diabetes is diagnosed based on plasma glucose values measured during the OGTT. Glucose levels are normally lower during pregnancy, so the threshold values for diagnosis of diabetes in pregnancy are lower. If a woman has two plasma glucose values meeting or exceeding any of the following numbers, she has gestational diabetes: a fasting plasma glucose level of 95 mg/dL, a 1-hour level of 180 mg/dL, a 2-hour level of 155 mg/dL, or a 3-hour level of 140 mg/dL.

What are the other forms of impaired glucose metabolism (also called pre-diabetes)?

People with pre-diabetes, a state between "normal" and "diabetes," are at risk for developing diabetes, heart attacks, and strokes. However, studies suggest that weight loss and increased physical activity can prevent or delay diabetes. There are two forms of pre-diabetes.

Impaired Fasting Glucose: A person has impaired fasting glucose (IFG) when fasting plasma glucose is 100 to 125 mg/dL. This level is higher than normal but less than the level indicating a diagnosis of diabetes.

Impaired Glucose Tolerance: Impaired glucose tolerance (IGT) means that blood glucose during the oral glucose tolerance test is higher than normal but not high enough for a diagnosis of diabetes. IGT is diagnosed when the glucose level is 140 to 199 mg/dL 2 hours after a person drinks a liquid containing 75 grams of glucose.

About 35 million people ages 40 to 74 have impaired fasting glucose and 16 million have impaired glucose tolerance. Because some people have both conditions, the total number of U.S. adults ages 40 to 74 with pre-diabetes comes to about 41 million. These recent estimates were calculated using data from the 1988–1994 National Health and Nutrition Examination Survey and projected to the 2000 U.S. population.

What are the scope and impact of diabetes?

Diabetes is widely recognized as one of the leading causes of death and disability in the United States. In 2000, it was the sixth leading cause of death. However, diabetes is likely to be underreported as the underlying cause of death on death certificates. About 65 percent of deaths among those with diabetes are attributed to heart disease and stroke.

Diabetes is associated with long-term complications that affect almost every part of the body. The disease often leads to blindness, heart and blood vessel disease, stroke, kidney failure, amputations, and nerve damage. Uncontrolled diabetes can complicate pregnancy, and birth defects are more common in babies born to women with diabetes.

In 2002, diabetes cost the United States $132 billion. Indirect costs, including disability payments, time lost from work, and premature death, totaled $40 billion; direct medical costs for diabetes care, including hospitalizations, medical care, and treatment supplies, totaled $92 billion.

Who gets diabetes?

Diabetes is not contagious. People cannot catch it from each other. However, certain factors can increase the risk of developing diabetes.

Type 1 diabetes occurs equally among males and females, but is more common in whites than in nonwhites. Data from the World Health Organization's Multinational Project for Childhood Diabetes indicate that type 1 diabetes is rare in most African, American Indian, and Asian populations. However, some northern European countries, including Finland and Sweden, have high rates of type 1 diabetes. The reasons for these differences are unknown.

Type 2 diabetes is more common in older people, especially in people who are overweight, and occurs more often in African Americans, American Indians, some Asian Americans, Native Hawaiians and other Pacific Islander Americans, and Hispanic Americans. On average, non-Hispanic African Americans are 1.6 times as likely to have diabetes as non-Hispanic whites of the same age. Hispanic Americans are 1.5 times as likely to have diabetes as non-Hispanic whites of similar age. American Indians have one of the highest rates of diabetes in the world. On average, American Indians and Alaska

Natives are 2.2 times as likely to have diabetes as non-Hispanic whites of similar age. Although prevalence data for diabetes among Asian Americans and Pacific Islanders are limited, some groups, such as Native Hawaiians and Japanese and Filipino residents of Hawaii aged 20 or older, are about twice as likely to have diabetes as white residents of Hawaii of similar age.

The prevalence of diabetes in the United States is likely to increase for several reasons. First, a large segment of the population is aging. Also, Hispanic Americans and other minority groups make up the fastest-growing segment of the U.S. population. Finally, Americans are increasingly overweight and sedentary. According to recent estimates, the prevalence of diabetes in the United States is predicted to reach 8.9 percent of the population by 2025.

✎ **What's It Mean?**

Coma: A state of profound unconsciousness caused by disease, injury, or poison. [1]

Hormone: Chemicals produced by glands in the body and circulated in the bloodstream. Hormones control the actions of certain cells or organs. [1]

Kidney: Body organ that filters blood for the secretion of urine. [1]

Plasma: The clear, yellowish, fluid part of the blood that carries the blood cells. [2]

Stroke: In medicine, a loss of blood flow to part of the brain, which damages brain tissue. Strokes are caused by blood clots and broken blood vessels in the brain. Symptoms include dizziness, numbness, weakness on one side of the body, and problems with talking, writing, or understanding language. The risk of stroke is increased by high blood pressure, older age, smoking, diabetes, high cholesterol, heart disease, atherosclerosis (a build-up of fatty material and plaque inside the coronary arteries), and a family history of stroke. [2]

Virus: A microorganism that can infect cells and cause disease. [1]

Source: [1] "Genetics Home Reference Glossary," a service of the U.S. National Library of Medicine, July 2005; available at http://www.ghr.nlm.nih.gov. [2] "Dictionary of Cancer Terms," National Cancer Institute, cited July 2005; available at http://www.cancer.gov.

How is diabetes managed?

Before the discovery of insulin in 1921, everyone with type 1 diabetes died within a few years after diagnosis. Although insulin is not considered a cure, its discovery was the first major breakthrough in diabetes treatment.

Today, healthy eating, physical activity, and taking insulin via injection or an insulin pump are the basic therapies for type 1 diabetes. The amount of insulin must be balanced with food intake and daily activities. Blood glucose levels must be closely monitored through frequent blood glucose checking.

Healthy eating, physical activity, and blood glucose testing are the basic management tools for type 2 diabetes. In addition, many people with type 2 diabetes require oral medication, insulin, or both to control their blood glucose levels.

People with diabetes must take responsibility for their day-to-day care. Much of the daily care involves keeping blood glucose levels from going too low or too high. When blood glucose levels drop too low—a condition known as hypoglycemia—a person can become nervous, shaky, and confused. Judgment can be impaired, and if blood glucose falls too low, fainting can occur.

A person can also become ill if blood glucose levels rise too high, a condition known as hyperglycemia.

People with diabetes should see a health care provider who will help them learn to manage their diabetes and who will monitor their diabetes control. An endocrinologist is a doctor who often specializes in diabetes care. In addition, people with diabetes often see ophthalmologists for eye examinations, podiatrists for routine foot care, and dietitians and diabetes educators to learn the skills needed for day-to-day diabetes management.

Chapter 2

Type 1 Diabetes

After school, when her friends flock to the store to pig out on candy and snack cakes, Sara passes up the sugary treats and sticks to the bottled water and half of a sandwich she packs. Her friends sometimes tease her about her self-control, but they don't know that Sara has diabetes (pronounced: dye-uh-be-tees). Watching what she eats, getting plenty of exercise, and taking special medicine helps Sara live a normal, healthy life.

What is diabetes?

Diabetes is a disease that affects how the body uses glucose (pronounced: gloo-kose), a sugar that is the body's main source of fuel. Like a car needs gasoline, your body needs glucose to keep running. Here's how it should work.

1. You eat.

2. Glucose from the food enters your bloodstream.

3. Your pancreas makes a hormone called insulin (pronounced: in-suh-lin).

4. Insulin helps the glucose get into the body's cells.

5. Your body gets the energy it needs.

About This Chapter: Reprinted from "Type 1 Diabetes: What Is It?" This information was provided by TeensHealth, one of the largest resources online for medically reviewed health information written for parents, kids, and teens. For more articles like this one, visit www.TeensHealth.org, or www.KidsHealth.org. © 2005 The Nemours Center for Children's Health Media, a division of The Nemours Foundation.

The pancreas is a long, flat gland in your belly that helps your body digest food. It also makes insulin. Insulin is kind of like a key that opens the doors to the cells of the body. It lets the glucose in. Then the glucose can move out of the blood and into the cells.

But if someone has diabetes, the body either can't make insulin or the insulin doesn't work in the body like it should. The glucose can't get into the cells normally, so the blood sugar level gets too high. Lots of sugar in the blood makes people sick if they don't get treatment.

What is type 1 diabetes?

There are two major types of diabetes: type 1 and type 2. Each type causes high blood sugar levels in a different way.

In type 1 diabetes (which used to be called insulin-dependent diabetes or juvenile diabetes), the pancreas can't make insulin. That's because—for some reason doctors don't completely understand—the body's immune system attacked the pancreas and destroyed the cells that make insulin.

> ♣ **It's A Fact!!**
> Once a person has type 1 diabetes, the pancreas can't ever make insulin again. To fix this problem, someone who has type 1 diabetes needs to take insulin through regular shots or an insulin pump.

When a person has type 1 diabetes, the body is still able to get glucose from food, but the lack of insulin means that glucose can't get into the cells where it's needed. So the glucose stays in the blood. This makes the blood sugar level very high and causes health problems.

Type 2 diabetes is different from type 1 diabetes. In type 2 diabetes, the pancreas still makes insulin. But the insulin doesn't work in the body like it should and blood sugar levels get too high.

What causes type 1 diabetes?

No one knows for sure what causes type 1 diabetes, but scientists think it has something to do with genes. Genes are like instructions for how the body should look and work that are passed on by parents to their kids. But just getting the genes for diabetes isn't usually enough. In most cases, something else has to happen—like getting a virus infection—for a person to get type 1 diabetes.

Type 1 diabetes can't be prevented. Doctors can't even tell who will get it and who won't.

How do people know if they have it?

People can have diabetes without knowing it because the symptoms aren't always obvious, and they can take a long time to develop. Type 1 diabetes may come on gradually or suddenly.

When a person first has type 1 diabetes, he or she may:

- pee a lot because the body tries to get rid of the extra blood sugar by passing it out of the body in the urine.

- drink a lot to make up for all that peeing.

- eat a lot because the body is hungry for the energy it can't get from sugar.

- lose weight because the body starts to use fat and muscle for fuel.

- feel tired all the time.

Also, girls who have developed diabetes are more likely to get vaginal yeast infections before they're diagnosed and treated.

If these early symptoms of diabetes aren't recognized and treatment isn't started, chemicals can build up in the blood and cause stomach pain, nausea, vomiting, breathing problems, and even loss of consciousness. Doctors call this diabetic ketoacidosis, or DKA.

There's good news, though—getting treatment can control or stop these diabetes symptoms from happening and reduce the risk of long-term problems. Doctors can say for sure if a person has diabetes by testing urine and blood samples for glucose. If the doctor suspects that a kid or teen has diabetes, he or she may send the person to see a pediatric endocrinologist (pronounced: pee-dee-ah-trik en-doh-krih-nah-leh-jist)—a doctor who specializes in diagnosing and treating children and teens living with diseases of the endocrine system, such as diabetes and growth problems.

Living With Type 1 Diabetes

People with type 1 diabetes have to pay a little more attention to what they're eating and doing than people who don't have diabetes. They need to:

- check blood sugar levels a few times a day by testing a small blood sample.

- give themselves insulin injections or use an insulin pump.

- eat a balanced, healthy diet and pay special attention to the amounts of sugars and starches in the food they eat and the timing of their meals.

- get regular exercise to help control blood sugar levels and help avoid some of the long-term health problems that diabetes can cause, like heart disease.

- have regular checkups with doctors and other people on their diabetes health care team so they can stay healthy and get treatment for any diabetes problems.

Sometimes people who have diabetes feel different from their friends because they need to take insulin, think about how they eat, and control their blood sugar levels every day. And some people with diabetes want to deny that they even have it. They might hope that if they ignore diabetes, it will just go away. They may feel angry, depressed, helpless, or that their parents are constantly in their faces about their diabetes management.

Diabetes brings challenges, of course. But people with diabetes play sports, travel, date, go to school, and work just like their friends. There are thousands of teens with diabetes, all learning to handle the same challenges.

✔ Quick Tip

If you've been diagnosed with diabetes, it's normal to feel like your world has been turned upside down. Fortunately, your doctor or diabetes care team is there to provide answers and support. Don't hesitate to ask your doctors, dietitian, and other health professionals for advice and tips. There are also support groups where you can talk about your feelings and find out how other people cope with the disease.

Chapter 3

Type 2 Diabetes

What is type 2 diabetes?

Diabetes is a disease in which blood glucose levels are above normal. People with diabetes have problems converting food to energy. After a meal, food is broken down into a sugar called glucose, which is carried by the blood to cells throughout the body. Cells use the hormone insulin, made in the pancreas, to help them process blood glucose into energy.

People develop type 2 diabetes because the cells in the muscles, liver, and fat do not use insulin properly. Eventually, the pancreas cannot make enough insulin for the body's needs. As a result, the amount of glucose in the blood increases while the cells are starved of energy. Over the years, high blood glucose damages nerves and blood vessels, leading to complications such as heart disease, stroke, blindness, kidney disease, nerve problems, gum infections, and amputation.

How can type 2 diabetes be prevented?

Although people with diabetes can prevent or delay complications by keeping blood glucose levels close to normal, preventing or delaying the

About This Chapter: Excerpted from "Am I at Risk for Type 2 Diabetes?," a publication of the National Diabetes Information Clearinghouse (NDIC), a service of the National Institute of Diabetes and Digestive and Kidney Diseases (NIDDK), National Institutes of Health (NIH), NIH Publication No. 04-4805, April 2004.

development of type 2 diabetes in the first place is even better. The results of a major federally funded study, the Diabetes Prevention Program (DPP), show how to do so.

This study of 3,234 people at high risk for diabetes showed that moderate diet and exercise resulting in a 5- to 7-percent weight loss could delay and possibly prevent type 2 diabetes.

Study participants were overweight and had higher than normal levels of blood glucose, a condition called pre-diabetes (impaired glucose tolerance). Both pre-diabetes and obesity are strong risk factors for type 2 diabetes. Because of the high risk among some minority groups, about half of the DPP participants were African American, American Indian, Asian American, Pacific Islander, or Hispanic American/Latino.

The DPP tested two approaches to preventing diabetes: a healthy eating and exercise program (lifestyle changes), and the diabetes drug metformin. People in the lifestyle modification group exercised about 30 minutes a day 5 days a week (usually by walking) and lowered their intake of fat and calories. Those who took the diabetes drug metformin received standard information on exercise and diet. A third group received only standard information on exercise and diet.

The results showed that people in the lifestyle modification group reduced their risk of getting type 2 diabetes by 58 percent. Average weight loss in the first year of the study was 15 pounds. Lifestyle modification was even more effective in those 60 and older. They reduced their risk by 71 percent. People receiving metformin reduced their risk by 31 percent.

What are the signs and symptoms of type 2 diabetes?

Many people have no signs or symptoms. Symptoms can also be so mild that you might not even notice them.

Here is what to look for:

• Increased thirst

• Increased hunger

• Fatigue

♣ **It's A Fact!!**
More than five million people in the United States have type 2 diabetes and do not know it.

- Increased urination, especially at night

- Weight loss

- Blurred vision

- Sores that do not heal

☞ Remember!!
It is important to find out early if you have diabetes because treatment can prevent damage to the body from diabetes.

Sometimes people have symptoms but do not suspect diabetes. They delay scheduling a checkup because they do not feel sick. Many people do not find out they have the disease until they have diabetes complications, such as blurry vision or heart trouble.

Type 2 diabetes, formerly called adult-onset or noninsulin-dependent diabetes, is the most common form of diabetes. People can develop type 2 diabetes at any age, even during childhood. This form of diabetes usually begins with insulin resistance, a condition in which fat, muscle, and liver cells do not use insulin properly. At first, the pancreas keeps up with the added demand by producing more insulin. In time, however, it loses the ability to secrete enough insulin in response to meals. Being overweight and inactive increases the chances of developing type 2 diabetes. Treatment includes taking diabetes medicines, making wise food choices, exercising regularly, taking aspirin daily, and controlling blood pressure and cholesterol.

Besides age and overweight, what other factors increase my risk for type 2 diabetes?

To find out your risk for type 2 diabetes, see how many of the following items apply to you.

- I have a parent, brother, or sister with diabetes.

- My family background is African American, American Indian, Asian American, Pacific Islander, or Hispanic American/Latino.

- I have had gestational diabetes, or I gave birth to at least one baby weighing more than 9 pounds.

- My blood pressure is 140/90 or higher, or I have been told that I have high blood pressure.

- My cholesterol levels are not normal. My HDL cholesterol ("good" cholesterol) is 35 or lower, or my triglyceride level is 250 or higher.

- I am fairly inactive. I exercise less than three times a week.

What can I do about my risk?

You can do a lot to lower your chances of getting diabetes. Exercising regularly, reducing fat and calorie intake, and losing weight can all help you reduce your risk of developing type 2 diabetes. Lowering blood pressure and cholesterol levels also help you stay healthy.

If you are overweight, then take these steps:

- Reach and maintain a reasonable body weight.

- Make wise food choices most of the time.

- Be physically active every day.

If you are fairly inactive, be physically active every day.

If your blood pressure is 140/90 or higher, then take these steps:

- Reach and maintain a reasonable body weight.

- Make wise food choices most of the time.

- Reduce your intake of salt and alcohol.

- Be physically active every day.

> ✔ **Quick Tip**
> **Getting Started**
>
> Making big changes in your life is hard, especially if you are faced with more than one change. You can make it easier by taking these steps:
>
> - Make a plan to change behavior.
>
> - Decide exactly what you will do and when you will do it.
>
> - Plan what you need to get ready.
>
> - Think about what might prevent you from reaching your goals.
>
> - Find family and friends who will support and encourage you.
>
> - Decide how you will reward yourself when you do what you have planned.
>
> Your doctor, a dietitian, or a counselor can help you make a plan.

- Talk to your doctor about whether you need medicine to control your blood pressure.

  If your checked cholesterol levels are not normal, then take these steps:

- Make wise food choices most of the time.

- Be physically active every day.

- Talk to your doctor about whether you need medicine to control your cholesterol levels.

Chapter 4

Gestational Diabetes

What is gestational diabetes?

Gestational (jes-TAY-shun-ul) diabetes is diabetes that is found for the first time when a woman is pregnant. Diabetes means that blood glucose (also called blood sugar) is too high. The human body uses glucose for energy. But too much glucose in the blood can be harmful. When a woman is pregnant, too much glucose is not good for her baby.

What causes gestational diabetes?

Changing hormones and weight gain are part of a healthy pregnancy. But both changes make it hard for a woman's body to keep up with its need for a hormone called insulin. When that happens, her body doesn't get the energy it needs from the food she eats.

What is a woman's risk of gestational diabetes?

To learn risk for gestational diabetes, a woman should evaluate how many of the following items apply to her. She should talk with her doctor about her risk at her first prenatal visit.

About This Chapter: Excerpted from "What I Need to Know about Gestational Diabetes," a publication of the National Diabetes Information Clearinghouse (NDIC), a service of the National Institute of Diabetes and Digestive and Kidney Diseases (NIDDK), National Institutes of Health (NIH), NIH Publication No. 04-5129, April 2004.

- I have a parent, brother, or sister with diabetes.

- I am African American, American Indian, Asian American, Hispanic American, or Pacific Islander.

- I am 25 years old or older.

- I am overweight.

- I have had gestational diabetes before, or I have given birth to at least one baby weighing more than 9 pounds.

♣ **It's A Fact!!**
Out of every 100 pregnant women in the United States, three to eight get gestational diabetes.

- I have been told that I have "pre-diabetes," a condition in which blood glucose levels are higher than normal, but not yet high enough for a diagnosis of diabetes. Other names for it are "impaired glucose tolerance" and "impaired fasting glucose."

If any of these items apply to her, she should ask her health care team about testing for gestational diabetes.

- A woman is at high risk if she is very overweight, had gestational diabetes before, has a strong family history of diabetes, or has glucose in her urine.

- A woman is at average risk if one or more of the risk factors apply to her.

- A woman is at low risk if none of the risk factors apply to her.

When will a woman be checked for gestational diabetes?

Her doctor will decide when she needs to be checked for diabetes depending on her risk factors.

- If she is at high risk, her blood glucose level may be checked at her first prenatal visit. If her test results are normal, she will be checked again sometime between weeks 24 and 28 of her pregnancy.

- If she has an average risk for gestational diabetes, she will be tested sometime between weeks 24 and 28 of pregnancy.

- If she is at low risk, her doctor may decide that she does not need to be checked.

How is gestational diabetes diagnosed?

A woman's health care team will check her blood glucose level. Depending on her risk and her test results, she may have one or more of the following tests.

- Fasting Blood Glucose

- Random Blood Glucose

- Oral Glucose Tolerance

How will gestational diabetes affect a woman's baby?

Untreated or uncontrolled gestational diabetes can mean problems for a woman's baby, such as:

- being born very large and with extra fat; this can make delivery difficult and more dangerous for her baby.

- low blood glucose right after birth.

- breathing problems.

If she has gestational diabetes, her health care team may recommend some extra tests to check on her baby, such as:

- an ultrasound exam, to see how the baby is growing.

- "kick counts" to check the baby's activity (the time between the baby's movements) or special stress tests.

Working closely with her health care team will help a woman give birth to a healthy baby.

How will gestational diabetes affect the mother?

Often, women with gestational diabetes have no symptoms. Gestational diabetes may:

- increase the risk of high blood pressure during pregnancy.

- increase the risk of a large baby and the need for cesarean section at delivery.

The good news is gestational diabetes will probably go away after the baby is born. However, a woman who has had gestational diabetes will be more likely to get type 2 diabetes later in life. She may also get gestational diabetes again if she gets pregnant again.

Some women wonder whether breast-feeding is OK after they have had gestational diabetes. Breast-feeding is recommended for most babies, including those whose mothers had gestational diabetes.

Gestational diabetes is serious, even if a woman has no symptoms. Taking care of herself helps keep the baby healthy.

How is gestational diabetes treated?

Treating gestational diabetes means taking steps to keep blood glucose levels in a target range. A pregnant woman will learn how to control her blood glucose using:

- a meal plan.
- physical activity.
- insulin (if needed).

After she has the baby, how can a woman find out whether her diabetes is gone?

She will probably have a blood glucose test 6 to 12 weeks after the baby is born to see whether she still has diabetes. For most women, gestational diabetes goes away after pregnancy. She is, however, at risk of having gestational diabetes during future pregnancies or getting type 2 diabetes later. Women who have had gestational diabetes should continue to be tested for diabetes or pre-diabetes every 3 years.

Chapter 5

Diabetes In African Americans

Today, diabetes mellitus is one of the most serious health challenges facing the United States. The following statistics illustrate the magnitude of this disease among African Americans.

- 2.8 million African Americans have diabetes.

- On average, African Americans are twice as likely to have diabetes as white Americans of similar age.

- Approximately 13 percent of all African Americans have diabetes.

- African Americans with diabetes are more likely to develop diabetes complications and experience greater disability from the complications than white Americans with diabetes.

- Death rates for people with diabetes are 27 percent higher for African Americans compared with whites.

Most African Americans (about 90 percent to 95 percent) with diabetes have type 2 diabetes. This type of diabetes usually develops in adults and is caused by the body's resistance to the action of insulin and to impaired insulin

About This Chapter: Excerpted from "Diabetes in African Americans," a publication of the National Diabetes Information Clearinghouse (NDIC), a service of the National Institute of Diabetes and Digestive and Kidney Diseases (NIDDK), National Institutes of Health (NIH), NIH Publication No. 02-3266, May 2002.

secretion. It can be treated with diet, exercise, diabetes pills, and injected insulin. A small number of African Americans (about 5 percent to 10 percent) have type 1 diabetes, which usually develops before age 20 and is always treated with insulin.

How many African Americans have diabetes?

The proportion of the African American population that has diabetes rises from less than 1 percent for those aged younger than 20 years to as high as 32 percent for women age 65–74 years. Overall, among those age 20 years or older, the rate is 11.8 percent for women and 8.5 percent for men.

> ♣ **It's A Fact!!**
> On average, African Americans are twice as likely to have diabetes as white Americans of similar age.

About one-third of total diabetes cases are undiagnosed among African Americans. This is similar to the proportion for other racial/ethnic groups in the United States.

National health surveys during the past 35 years show that the percentage of the African American population that has been diagnosed with diabetes is increasing dramatically. In 1976–80, total diabetes prevalence in African Americans ages 40 to 74 years was 8.9 percent; in 1988–94, total prevalence had increased to 18.2 percent—a doubling of the rate in just 12 years.

Prevalence in African Americans is much higher than in white Americans. Among those ages 40 to 74 years in a1988–94 survey, the rate was 11.2 percent for whites, but was 18.2 percent for African Americans.

What risk factors increase the chance of developing type 2 diabetes?

The frequency of diabetes in African American adults is influenced by the same risk factors that are associated with type 2 diabetes in other populations. Two categories of risk factors increase the chance of developing type 2 diabetes. The first is genetics. The second is medical and lifestyle risk factors, including impaired glucose tolerance, gestational diabetes, hyperinsulinemia and insulin resistance, obesity, and physical inactivity.

Genetic Risk Factors: The common finding that "diabetes runs in families" indicates that there is a strong genetic component to type 1 and type 2 diabetes. Many scientists are now conducting research to determine the genes that cause diabetes. For type 1 diabetes, certain genes related to immunology have been implicated. For type 2 diabetes, there seem to be diabetes genes that determine insulin secretion and insulin resistance. Some researchers believe that African Americans inherited a "thrifty gene" from their African ancestors. Years ago, this gene enabled Africans, during "feast and famine" cycles, to use food energy more efficiently when food was scarce. Today, with fewer such cycles, the thrifty gene that developed for survival may instead make the person more susceptible to developing type 2 diabetes.

Pre-diabetes (Impaired Glucose Tolerance And Impaired Fasting Glucose): In some people, blood glucose levels are higher than normal but not high enough for them to be diagnosed with diabetes. These individuals are described as having pre-diabetes, also called impaired glucose tolerance (IGT) or impaired fasting glucose (IFG). People with pre-diabetes are at higher risk of developing type 2 diabetes than people with normal glucose tolerance. Rates of IGT among adults ages 40 to 74 years are similar for African Americans (13 percent) and white (15 percent) Americans.

Gestational Diabetes (GDM): About 2 to 5 percent of pregnant women develop mild abnormalities in glucose levels and insulin secretion and are considered to have gestational diabetes. Although these women's glucose and insulin levels often return to normal after pregnancy, as many as 50 percent may develop type 2 diabetes within 20 years of the pregnancy.

Hyperinsulinemia And Insulin Resistance: Higher-than-normal levels of fasting insulin, called hyperinsulinemia, are associated with an increased risk of developing type 2 diabetes. Hyperinsulinemia often predates diabetes by several years. Among people who did not have diabetes in a survey, insulin levels were higher in African Americans than in whites, particularly African American women, indicating their greater predisposition for developing type 2 diabetes. Another study showed a higher rate of hyperinsulinemia in African American adolescents compared with white American adolescents.

Obesity: Overweight is a major risk factor for type 2 diabetes. Overweight is increasing in the United States, both in adolescents and in adults. Survey data shows that African American adults have substantially higher rates of obesity than white Americans.

In addition to the overall level of obesity, the location of the excess weight is also a risk factor for type 2 diabetes. Excess weight carried above the waist is a stronger risk factor than excess weight carried below the waist. African Americans have a greater tendency to develop upper-body obesity, which increases their risk of diabetes.

Although African Americans have higher rates of obesity, researchers do not believe that obesity alone accounts for their higher prevalence of diabetes. Even when compared with white Americans with the same levels of obesity, age, and socioeconomic status, African Americans still have higher rates of diabetes. Other factors, yet to be understood, appear to be responsible.

Physical Inactivity: Regular physical activity is a protective factor against type 2 diabetes and, conversely, lack of physical activity is a risk factor for developing diabetes. Researchers suspect that a lack of exercise is one factor contributing to the high rates of diabetes in African Americans. A survey indicated that 50 percent of African American men and 67 percent of African American women reported that they participated in little or no leisure time physical activity.

♣ It's A Fact!!

African American children seem to have lower rates of type 1 diabetes than white American children. Researchers tend to agree that genetics probably makes type 1 diabetes less common among children with African ancestry compared with children of European ancestry. However, recent reports indicate an increasing prevalence of type 2 diabetes in children, especially in those with African American, American Indian, or Hispanic family background.

✎ What's It Mean?

Blood Pressure: The force of the blood against the artery walls. Two levels of blood pressure are measured: the highest, or systolic, occurs when the heart pumps blood into the blood vessels, and the lowest, or diastolic, occurs when the heart rests. [1]

Hypertension: Abnormally high blood pressure. [2]

Lipids: Fatty substances, including simple fats, their major components (i.e., fatty acids), and various fat-soluble substances (e.g., cholesterol). [3]

Source: [1] "Publications and Products," "Take Charge of Your Diabetes," "Glossary," National Center for Chronic Disease Prevention and Health Promotions, Department of Health and Human Services, January 2005; available online at http://www.cdc.gov/diabetes/pubs/tcyd/appendix.htm. [2] "Genetics Home Reference Glossary," a service of the U.S. National Library of Medicine, July 2005; available at http://www.ghr.nlm.nih.gov. [3] "Glossary," National Institute on Alcohol Abuse and Alcoholism, October 2004; available online at http://www.niaaa.nih.gov/publications/arh27-4/331-332.htm.

How does diabetes affect African American women during pregnancy?

Gestational diabetes, in which blood glucose values are elevated above normal during pregnancy, occurs in about 2 percent to 5 percent of all pregnant women. Perinatal problems such as macrosomia (large body size) and neonatal hypoglycemia (low blood sugar) are higher in these pregnancies. The women generally return to normal glucose values after childbirth. However, once a woman has had gestational diabetes, she has an increased risk of developing gestational diabetes in future pregnancies. In addition, experts estimate that about half of women with gestational diabetes develop type 2 diabetes within 20 years of the pregnancy.

Several studies have shown that the occurrence of gestational diabetes in African American women may be 50 percent to 80 percent more frequent than in white women.

How do diabetes complications affect African Americans?

Compared with white Americans, African Americans experience higher rates of diabetes complications such as eye disease, kidney failure, and amputations. They also experience greater disability from these complications.

Proper diabetes management can influence some factors that influence the frequency of these complications, such as high blood glucose levels, abnormal blood lipids, high blood pressure, and cigarette smoking.

Eye Disease: Diabetic retinopathy is a deterioration of the blood vessels in the eye that is caused by high blood glucose. It can lead to impaired vision and, ultimately, to blindness. The frequency of diabetic retinopathy is 40 percent to 50 percent higher in African Americans than in white Americans. Retinopathy may also occur more frequently in African Americans than in whites because of their higher rate of hypertension. Although blindness caused by diabetic retinopathy is believed to be more frequent in African Americans than in whites, there are no valid studies that compare rates of blindness between the two groups.

Kidney Failure: African Americans with diabetes experience kidney failure, also called end-stage renal disease (ESRD), about four times more often than diabetic white Americans. In 1995, there were 27,258 new cases of ESRD attributed to diabetes in African Americans. Diabetes is the leading cause of kidney failure and accounted for 43 percent of the new cases of ESRD among African Americans during 1992–1996. Hypertension, the second leading cause of ESRD, accounted for 42 percent of cases. In spite of their high rates of ESRD, African Americans have better survival rates after they develop kidney failure than white Americans.

Amputations: Based on a U.S. hospital discharge survey, there were about 13,000 amputations among African American diabetic individuals in 1994, which involved 155,000 days in the hospital. African Americans with diabetes are much more likely to undergo a lower-extremity amputation than white or Hispanic Americans with diabetes. The hospitalization rate of amputations for African Americans was 9.3 per 1,000 patients in 1994, compared with 5.8 per 1,000 white diabetic patients. However, the average length of hospital stay was lower for African Americans (12.1 days) than for white Americans (16.5 days).

Does diabetes cause excess deaths in African Americans?

Diabetes was an uncommon cause of death among African Americans at the turn of the century. By 1994, however, death certificates listed diabetes as the seventh leading cause of death for African Americans. For those age 45 years or older, it was the fifth leading cause of death.

Chapter 6

Diabetes In Hispanic Americans

Diabetes in Hispanic Americans is a serious health challenge because of the increased prevalence of diabetes in this population, the greater number of risk factors for diabetes in Hispanics, the greater incidence of several diabetes complications, and the growing number of people of Hispanic ethnicity in the United States.

The following statistics illustrate the magnitude of diabetes among Hispanic Americans:

- In 2000, of the 30 million Hispanic Americans, about 2 million had been diagnosed with diabetes.

- About 10.2 percent of all Hispanic Americans have diabetes.

- On average, Hispanic Americans are 1.9 times more likely to have diabetes than non-Hispanic whites of similar age.

- Diabetes is particularly common among middle-aged and older Hispanic Americans. For those ages 50 or older, about 25 to 30 percent have either diagnosed or undiagnosed diabetes.

About This Chapter: Excerpted from "Diabetes in Hispanic Americans," a publication of the National Diabetes Information Clearinghouse (NDIC), a service of the National Institute of Diabetes and Digestive and Kidney Diseases (NIDDK), National Institutes of Health (NIH), NIH Publication No. 02-3265, May 2002.

- Diabetes is twice as common in Mexican American and Puerto Rican adults as in non-Hispanic whites. The prevalence of diabetes in Cuban Americans is lower, but still higher than that of non-Hispanic whites.

- As in all populations, having risk factors for diabetes increases the chance that a Hispanic American will develop diabetes. Risk factors seem to be more common among Hispanics than non-Hispanic whites. These factors include a family history of diabetes, gestational diabetes, impaired glucose tolerance, hyperinsulinemia and insulin resistance, obesity, and physical inactivity.

- Higher rates of the diabetes complications nephropathy (kidney disease), retinopathy (eye disease), and peripheral vascular disease have been documented in studies of Mexican Americans, whereas lower rates of myocardial infarctions (heart attacks) have been found.

Most Hispanic Americans with diabetes (about 90 to 95 percent) have type 2 diabetes. This type of diabetes usually develops in adults and is caused by the body's resistance to the action of insulin and to impaired insulin secretion. It can be treated with diet, exercise, diabetes pills, and injected insulin. A small number of Hispanic Americans with diabetes (about 5 to 10 percent) have type 1 diabetes, which usually develops before age 20 and is always treated with insulin.

What major studies of diabetes have been done regarding Hispanic Americans?

Five population studies conducted in the past 20 years provide the majority of information that exists about the incidence and progression of diabetes among Hispanic Americans. The five studies are briefly described below:

- The Starr County Study (Texas), conducted in 1981, assessed the prevalence of severe hyperglycemia (high blood glucose levels) in almost 2,500 people ages 15 or older.

- The San Antonio Heart Study (Texas), begun in 1979 and still being conducted, assessed diabetes in more than 3,000 Mexican Americans and almost 2,000 non-Hispanic whites between the ages of 25 and 64.

- The San Luis Valley Diabetes Study (Colorado), a continuing study that began in 1984, estimated the prevalence of diabetes in Hispanics and non-Hispanic whites in two counties in southern Colorado.

- The Hispanic Health and Nutrition Examination Survey (HHANES), 1982–84, investigated the prevalence of diabetes in national samples of the three major Hispanic subgroups—Mexican Americans in the southwestern United States, Puerto Ricans in the New York City area, and Cuban Americans in south Florida. Approximately 6,600 people participated.

- The Third National Health and Nutrition Examination Survey (NHANES III), 1988–94, determined the prevalence and characteristics of people with diabetes in national samples of African Americans, Mexican Americans, and whites. Approximately 18,000 adults participated.

How many Hispanic Americans have diabetes?

Hispanic Americans are the second-largest and fastest growing minority group in the United States. In 1998, there were 30 million Hispanics in the United States, representing 11 percent of the population. By the year 2050, it is estimated that Hispanics will number 97 million and constitute 25 percent of the U.S. population.

Mexican Americans represent the largest Hispanic American subgroup, with 64.3 percent of the Hispanic population. Central and South Americans represent the second-largest Hispanic American subgroup, with 13.4 percent of the Hispanic population. The majority of Hispanic Americans live in the south-central and southwestern United States.

The proportion of the Mexican American population that has diabetes (defined by medical history or fasting plasma glucose of 126 mg/dL or greater) rises from less than 1 percent for those younger than 20 to as high as 33 percent for women ages 60 to 74. In almost every age group, prevalence is higher among women than men.

About one-third of total diabetes among Hispanic Americans is undiagnosed. This is similar to the proportion for other racial/ethnic groups in the United States.

Prevalence in Hispanic Americans is much higher than in Americans without Hispanic ancestry. Among those ages 40 to 74 in the 1988–94 survey, the rate was 11.2 percent for non-Hispanic whites, but 20.3 percent for Mexican Americans.

What factors increase the chance of developing type 2 diabetes?

The frequency of diabetes in Hispanic American adults is influenced by the same risk factors that are associated with type 2 diabetes in other populations. Two categories of risk factors increase the chance of developing type 2 diabetes. The first is genetics. The second comprises medical and lifestyle risk factors, including prediabetes, gestational diabetes, hyperinsulinemia and insulin resistance, obesity, and physical inactivity.

Genetic Risk Factors: A family history of diabetes increases the chance that people will develop diabetes. The San Antonio Heart Study showed that the prevalence of diabetes among Mexican Americans who have first-degree relatives (e.g., parents) with diabetes was twice as great as for those with no family history of diabetes.

Having American Indian or African genes (populations with a high prevalence of diabetes) is also thought to be a factor that causes the higher rates of diabetes in Hispanics. Hispanics, like all populations, inherit their susceptibility to diabetes from their ancestors. Hispanics have three groups of ancestors—Spaniards, American Indians, and Africans. Both American Indians and Africans have high rates of diabetes.

Although Cuban Americans have both American Indian and African ancestry, neither of these genetic roots contributes more than 20 percent to the current Cuban American gene pool. This may partly explain why Cuban Americans have a higher prevalence of type 2 diabetes than non-Hispanic white Americans, although not as high as the other Hispanic groups.

Pre-Diabetes (Impaired Glucose Tolerance And Impaired Fasting Glucose): In some people, the blood glucose level is higher than normal, but not enough to be diagnosed as diabetes. These individuals are described as having pre-diabetes. People with pre-diabetes are at higher risk of developing type 2 diabetes than people with normal glucose tolerance. Rates of impaired glucose tolerance among adults ages 40 to 74 in the NHANES III survey were higher for Mexican Americans (19 percent) than for non-Hispanic white Americans (15 percent).

Gestational Diabetes: About 2 to 5 percent of pregnant women in the United States develop mild abnormalities in glucose levels, insulin secretion, and insulin resistance and are considered to have gestational diabetes. Although these women's glucose and insulin levels often return to normal after pregnancy, as many as 50 percent may develop type 2 diabetes within 20 years of the pregnancy. Mexican American women may be at particularly high risk for developing type 2 diabetes. One study of 666 women with gestational diabetes in southern California found that each year an average of 12 percent developed type 2 diabetes after pregnancy.

Hyperinsulinemia And Insulin Resistance: Hyperinsulinemia (higher than normal levels of fasting insulin) and insulin resistance (an inability to use the body's own insulin to properly control blood glucose) are both hallmarks of an increased risk for developing type 2 diabetes. Hyperinsulinemia often predates diabetes by several years. Among people in the NHANES III survey who did not have diabetes, insulin levels were higher in Mexican Americans than in non-Hispanic whites, indicating their greater predisposition for developing type 2 diabetes. Several other studies have also shown a higher rate of hyperinsulinemia in Hispanics than in non-Hispanics.

Obesity: Obesity is a major risk factor for type 2 diabetes. Many racial/ethnic groups in the United States have high rates of obesity, and surveys show that obesity is increasing. Hispanics are more likely than non-Hispanic whites to be overweight. Mexican American adults, particularly women, have substantially higher rates of obesity than non-Hispanic white Americans, but rates that are similar to those of African Americans.

The degree to which obesity is a risk factor for diabetes depends not just on overall weight, but also on the location of the excess weight. Central or upper-body obesity is a stronger risk factor for type 2 diabetes than excess weight carried below the waist. Mexican Americans with upper body obesity have an increased risk of type 2 diabetes.

Physical Inactivity: Regular physical activity is a protective factor against type 2 diabetes and, conversely, lack of physical activity is a risk factor for developing diabetes. Researchers suspect that a lack of exercise is one factor contributing to the high rates of diabetes in Hispanic Americans. In the NHANES III survey, 65 percent of Mexican American men and 74 percent of Mexican American women reported that they participated in little or no leisure-time physical activity.

HHANES data showed that fewer men with high levels of work-related physical activity had diabetes. The San Antonio Heart Study also found that decreased leisure-time physical activity was related to a higher incidence of diabetes.

> **♣ It's A Fact!!**
> Recent reports indicate an increase in the prevalence of type 2 diabetes among Mexican American youth, especially among those who are overweight.

How does diabetes affect Hispanic young people?

Mexican American children in Colorado had lower rates of type 1 diabetes than non-Hispanic white children. However, the incidence of type 1 diabetes in Puerto Rican children in Philadelphia was similar to that of white children. Genetic, immunologic, and environmental factors are thought to be involved in the development of type 1 diabetes.

How does diabetes affect Hispanic women during pregnancy?

Gestational diabetes, in which blood glucose levels are elevated above normal during pregnancy, occurs in about 2 to 5 percent of all pregnant women. Perinatal problems such as macrosomia (large body size) and neonatal hypoglycemia (low blood sugar) are higher in these pregnancies. The women generally return to normal glucose levels after childbirth. Mexican American women, especially when they are overweight, have higher rates of gestational diabetes than non-Hispanic white women.

Once a woman has had gestational diabetes, she has an increased risk of developing gestational diabetes in future pregnancies.

In addition, experts estimate that about half of women with gestational diabetes develop type 2 diabetes within 20 years of the pregnancy. For Mexican American women, this may be as great as 12 percent per year.

How do diabetes complications affect Hispanic Americans?

Eye Disease: Diabetic retinopathy is a deterioration of the blood vessels in the eye that is caused by high blood glucose. It can lead to impaired vision and, ultimately, to blindness. In the San Antonio Heart Study, the rate of diabetic retinopathy among Mexican Americans was more than twice that of non-Hispanic white Americans. NHANES III also found that Mexican Americans had a two-fold higher rate of diabetic retinopathy. However, the San Luis Valley Diabetes Study found lower rates of retinopathy in Hispanics than in non-Hispanic whites.

The results of all three studies showed that the severity of the diabetes— as indicated by insulin use, higher glucose levels, and more years since diagnosis—was significantly associated with retinopathy.

Kidney Disease: Diabetes is the leading cause of kidney failure (nephropathy) in the United States. The San Antonio Heart Study showed that the prevalence of clinical evidence of kidney damage (proteinuria) was more frequent in Mexican Americans with diabetes than in non-Hispanic whites.

A higher incidence of protein in the urine (microalbuminuria), an early indicator of diabetic nephropathy, was also seen in the San Antonio Heart Study comparing Mexican Americans with non-Hispanic whites. However, the San Luis Valley Diabetes Study showed no difference between Hispanics and non-Hispanic whites in the incidence of diabetic nephropathy.

Mexican Americans who develop kidney failure fare better than many others on dialysis. According to a report from Texas, Mexican Americans survived longer on renal dialysis than non-Hispanic white Americans.

Nerve Disease: In the San Luis Valley Diabetes Study, there was no significant difference in the prevalence of diabetic neuropathy (nerve disease) between Hispanics and non-Hispanic whites. However, in the 1989 National Health Interview Survey, symptoms of sensory neuropathy were reported more frequently by Mexican Americans than by non-Hispanic whites or African Americans.

Peripheral Vascular Disease: In the San Antonio Heart Study, Mexican Americans with type 2 diabetes had a higher rate of peripheral vascular disease than non-Hispanic whites; however, this increased incidence was not statistically significant.

Heart Disease: Heart disease is the most common cause of death in people with both type 1 and type 2 diabetes. However, in the Texas and Colorado studies, Mexican Americans had lower rates of myocardial infarctions (heart attacks) than non-Hispanic white Americans.

✎ What's It Mean?

Immunologic: Relating to the immune system. [1]

Perinatal: Events that occur at or around the time of birth. [2]

Peripheral Vascular Disease: A common disorder in which the arteries supplying oxygen rich blood from the heart to a limb (typically one or both legs) are blocked. As a result, the organs do not get enough blood flow for normal function. [3]

Source: [1] Editor. [2] "HIV Glossary," AIDS info, a service of the U.S. Department of Health and Human Services, September 2002; available at http://www.aidsinfo.nih.gov/ed%5Fresources/glossary. [3] "NWHIC Web Site Glossary," U.S. Department of Health and Human Services, Office on Women's Health, cited July 2005; available at http://www.4woman.gov/Glossary.

Chapter 7

Diabetes In Asian And Pacific Islander Americans

Diabetes mellitus poses a rapidly growing health challenge to Asian and Pacific Islander Americans in the United States. In 1997, the Asian and Pacific Islander American (APIA) population was estimated to be about 10 million, almost a 50 percent increase since the 1990 census and representing about 3.8 percent of the total U.S. population. This group includes people whose origins are in the Far East, Southeast Asia, the Indian subcontinent, and the Pacific Islands. Results of the 1990 census showed that the APIA population had the greatest increase of any major ethnic group, doubling in size since the 1980 census. The Immigration Act of 1965 and the arrival of many Southeast Asian refugees under the Refugee Resettlement Program after 1975 contributed to the increase in population observed in the past two decades.

Asian and Pacific Islander Americans in the United States were classified into 28 Asian and 19 Pacific Islander ethnic groups for the 1990 U.S. census. These populations include people whose families originated in a variety of countries, providing great diversity in language, culture, and beliefs.

About This Chapter: Excerpted from "Diabetes in Asian and Pacific Islander Americans," a publication of the National Diabetes Information Clearinghouse (NDIC), a service of the National Institute of Diabetes and Digestive and Kidney Diseases (NIDDK), National Institutes of Health (NIH), NIH Publication No. 02-4667, May 2002.

Nearly 75 percent are foreign-born, but other members of this group are fifth-generation Asian-Americans.

The 1990 census showed that 56 percent of the APIA population lived in the western states. Seventy-three percent were located within seven states: California, Hawaii, Illinois, New Jersey, New York, Texas, and Washington.

Most Asian and Pacific Islander Americans with diabetes have type 2 diabetes. This type usually develops in adults, but it can also develop in children or adolescents. It is caused by the body's resistance to the action of insulin and by impaired insulin secretion. It can be managed with healthy eating, physical activity, oral diabetes medications, and/or injected insulin. Until recently, type 2 diabetes was rarely diagnosed in children and adolescents. However, recent reports highlight an increasing incidence of type 2 diabetes in children and adolescents. A small number of Asian and Pacific Islander Americans have type 1 diabetes, which usually develops before age 20 and is managed with insulin, healthy eating, and physical activity.

How many Asian and Pacific Islander Americans have diabetes?

Type 2 Diabetes: Prevalence data for Asian and Pacific Islander Americans are limited, but studies have shown that some groups within this population are at increased risk for developing type 2 diabetes compared with non-Hispanic white people in the United States.

A study of the prevalence of diabetes and glucose intolerance was conducted among Native Hawaiians in two rural communities. Results showed a 22.4 percent age-standardized prevalence of type 2 diabetes in people ages 30 or older. Prevalence was highest in people ages 60 to 64, who had a rate of 40 percent. This prevalence was four times higher than that of the non-Hispanic white population surveyed in the U.S. National Health and Nutrition Examination Survey II. Analysis of data collected in Hawaii from 1996 to 2000 showed that Native Hawaiians were 2.5 times more likely to have diabetes than non-Hispanic white residents of similar age.

In contrast, the prevalence of diabetes in some isolated Polynesian groups is relatively low. For example, in 1976 in Funafuti, Tuvalu, the prevalence was 1.1 percent in men and 7.2 percent in women. Researchers attributed

♣ It's A Fact!!

Studies of Japanese school children in Japan show a dramatic increase in the incidence of type 2 diabetes. Junior high age children had an incidence of 13.9 per 100,000, which was nearly 7 times the rate of type 1 diabetes in the same group.

the difference in rates to differences in physical activity. In that community, men were engaged in manual labor, but women were sedentary and consumed more calories than needed for their level of activity.

In Western Samoa, diabetes prevalence in a rural community (3.4 percent) was less than half the rate in an urban setting (7.8 percent), even after adjusting for body weight. Rural residents were much more active physically than their urban counterparts.

Recent reports in the literature highlight an increasing incidence of type 2 diabetes in youth, particularly in members of minority groups. Data about APIA youth are scarce, but trends among Asian youth may indicate future trends in the larger group. For example, studies of Japanese school children in Japan show a dramatic increase in the incidence of type 2 diabetes. Incidence in 1976 was 0.2 per 100,000 children; incidence in 1995 was 7.3 per 100,000. Junior high age children had an incidence of 13.9 per 100,000, which was nearly 7 times the rate of type 1 diabetes in the same group. Researchers attribute the increase in incidence to changes in food habits and rising rates of obesity.

Type 1 Diabetes: Type 1 diabetes in Asian children is relatively rare; rates are significantly lower than those among non-Hispanic whites. Data from one study suggested that environmental factors might be involved in the etiology of type 1 diabetes, since rates in Japanese children in Hawaii were higher than rates of type 1 diabetes in Japanese children in Tokyo.

What risk factors increase the chance that Asian and Pacific Islander Americans will develop type 2 diabetes?

Two categories of risk factors increase the chance of type 2 diabetes. The first is genetics. The second is medical and lifestyle factors, including obesity, diet, and physical inactivity. Individuals with impaired glucose tolerance, impaired fasting glucose, or insulin resistance are at higher risk of progressing to diabetes.

Genetic Risk Factors: Genetic background is a determining factor in the prevalence of type 2 diabetes. Few data exist on specific genetic causes in the APIA population, but some researchers have suggested that the "thrifty gene" theory may be involved in the increased prevalence of diabetes in some minority populations, particularly those with high rates of obesity. The thrifty gene theory, first proposed in 1962, suggests that population groups that experienced alternating periods of feast and famine gradually adapted by developing a way to store fat more efficiently during periods of plenty to better survive famines.

Obesity: Obesity is a major risk factor for type 2 diabetes among all races and ethnic groups. The degree to which obesity is a risk factor for diabetes depends not just on overall weight, but also on the location of the excess weight. Central or upper-body obesity is a stronger risk factor for type 2 diabetes than excess weight carried below the waist. In a study comparing Japanese people in Japan with Japanese people who had immigrated to Hawaii, the Hawaiian Japanese had a higher rate of obesity and double the prevalence of type 2 diabetes. The sharp increase in type 2 diabetes in youth has paralleled the dramatic increase of obesity in youth.

Diet And Physical Inactivity: As a result of migration and modernization, the food choices of some members of APIA subgroups have changed. Many of the APIA populations have abandoned a traditional plant- and fish-based diet and are choosing foods with more animal protein, animal fats, and processed carbohydrates. One study compared the dietary content of similarly aged Japanese-American men living in Seattle, Washington, with that of Japanese men in Japan. The Japanese-American diet was higher in calories, protein, fat, and carbohydrates. The mean daily intake of fat in Japanese-American men was 32.4 grams, in contrast to a mean intake of only 16.7 grams of fat in Japanese men. Other studies have shown that, for many Asian Americans, their diet in America is higher in calories and fat and lower in fiber than in their countries of origin.

Most studies have shown lower rates of physical activity in minorities than in non-Hispanic whites in the United States. With the increase in migration and urbanization, physical activity has been greatly reduced in the APIA population. Urbanization has caused this population to change from a lifestyle characterized by hard labor to a more sedentary one.

Findings in a study of 8,000 Japanese-American men living in Hawaii suggested that a Japanese lifestyle was associated with a reduced prevalence of type 2 diabetes. Components of this lifestyle included higher levels of physical activity and consumption of more carbohydrates and less fat and animal protein.

Pre-Diabetes (Impaired Glucose Tolerance And Impaired Fasting Glucose): Recent recommendations describe two categories of the physiological state between normal blood glucose and the diabetic range of blood glucose. Individuals are described as having impaired glucose tolerance (a 2-hour glucose value of between 140 and 199 mg/dL during the oral glucose tolerance test) or impaired fasting glucose (a fasting plasma glucose value of between 110 and 125 mg/dL).

Asian Americans have shown higher rates of impaired glucose tolerance than have non-Hispanic whites in a number of studies. The prevalence of impaired glucose tolerance among Native Hawaiians in one study was 15.6 percent; prevalence rates were constant across age groups.

Hyperinsulinemia And Insulin Resistance: Hyperinsulinemia (higher than normal levels of fasting insulin) and insulin resistance (the inability of the body to use its own insulin to properly control blood glucose) are both associated with an increased risk of developing type 2 diabetes. Hyperinsulinemia often predates diabetes by several years. These factors, possibly linked to the APIA population through genetics and obesity, increase the risk of developing type 2 diabetes.

How does diabetes affect Asian and Pacific Islander American women during pregnancy?

Gestational diabetes, in which blood glucose levels are elevated above normal during pregnancy, occurs in about 2 to 5 percent of all American pregnant women. Perinatal problems such as macrosomia (large body size) and neonatal hypoglycemia (low blood sugar) are higher in babies born to women with gestational diabetes. Although blood glucose levels generally return to normal after childbirth, an increased risk of developing gestational diabetes in future pregnancies remains. In addition, studies show that many women with gestational diabetes will develop type 2 diabetes later in life. Asian-American women seem to have rates of gestational diabetes that are similar to those of non-Hispanic white women in the United States.

✎ What's It Mean?

Coronary Artery Disease: Also called coronary heart disease. It is the most common type of heart disease that results from atherosclerosis—the gradual buildup of plaque in the coronary arteries, the blood vessels that bring blood to the heart. This disease develops slowly and silently, over decades. It can go virtually unnoticed until it produces a heart attack. [1]

Hypertension: Also known as high blood pressure. A cardiovascular disease, which means the blood vessels become tight and constricted, forcing your heart to pump harder to move blood through your body. These changes cause the blood to press on the vessel walls with greater force, which can damage blood vessels and organs, including the heart, kidneys, eyes, and brain. [1]

Ischemia: Decrease in the blood supply to an organ, tissue, or other part caused by the narrowing or blockage of the blood vessels. [1]

Perinatal: Events that occur at or around the time of birth. [2]

Stroke: Caused by a lack of blood flow to the brain, or bleeding in the brain. A person's speech, writing, balance, sensation, memory, thinking, attention, and learning are some of the areas that can be affected as a result of suffering a stroke. [1]

Source: [1] "NWHIC Web Site Glossary," U.S. Department of Health and Human Services, Office on Women's Health, cited July 2005; available at http://www.4woman.gov/Glossary. [2]"HIV Glossary," AIDS info, a service of the U.S. Department of Health and Human Services, September 2002; available at http://www.aidsinfo.nih.gov/ed%5Fresources/glossary.

How does diabetes affect cardiovascular health in Asian and Pacific Islander Americans?

Diabetes is a major risk factor for cardiovascular disease; data suggest that minorities in general have a rate of risk for this disease similar to that of the non-Hispanic white population. Both impaired glucose tolerance and type 2 diabetes were risk factors for coronary artery disease among Japanese Americans in a Seattle study. Although data on the relationship of stroke and hypertension to diabetes in this population are limited, ischemic heart disease is one of the leading causes of death for both men and women.

How do diabetes complications affect Asian and Pacific Islander Americans?

Diabetic Retinopathy: Diabetic retinopathy is a deterioration of the blood vessels in the eye caused by high blood glucose levels. It can lead to impaired vision and, ultimately, to blindness. In general, age-standardized rates of blindness from diabetes for nonwhites are double those for non-Hispanic whites. However, no data on Asian and Pacific Islander Americans are available.

Diabetic Nephropathy: Minority groups in general have higher rates of end-stage renal (kidney) disease related to diabetes than do non-Hispanic white people. Among the minority groups, Asian Americans and Pacific Islanders have the lowest prevalence of end-stage renal disease. Minorities have better survival rates after treatment with dialysis than do non-Hispanic white people.

Lower Extremity Amputation: There are no published reports on the rate of amputations among this population.

Does diabetes cause an inordinate number of deaths in Asian and Pacific Islander Americans?

Because mortality rates are based on the underlying cause of death on death certificates, the impact of diabetes on mortality among Asian and Pacific Islander Americans has been underestimated.

For APIA populations as a whole, diabetes ranked as the fifth highest cause on death certificates for people between 45 and 64. Among non-Hispanic whites, diabetes is the seventh leading cause of death. However, the age-adjusted mortality rate for Asian and Pacific Islander Americans from diabetes is 12.4 per 100,000, which falls below the rate of 15.9 per 100,000 for non-Hispanic white Americans. The APIA rate is well below rates for other minority populations (African American, 35.7; American Indian and Alaska Native, 30.3; and Hispanic American, 28.3).

A review of death records in American Samoa for the years 1962 to 1974 showed that the age-adjusted, diabetes-related mortality rate for Samoa was more than double that of the United States.

Chapter 8

Diabetes In American Indians And Alaska Natives

Diabetes mellitus is one of the most serious health challenges facing American Indians and Alaska Natives in the United States today. The disease is very common in many tribes, and morbidity and mortality from diabetes can be severe.

This population includes all people who derive their origins from any of the original peoples of North America and who continue to maintain cultural identification through tribal affiliations or community recognition. Great diversity in culture, language, location, lifestyles, and genetic heritage exists among American Indians and Alaska Natives. More than 500 Native American tribal organizations, with many differences in language and culture, exist in the United States.

In 1990, the U.S. Bureau of the Census used self-identification to classify people as part of this group. The American Indian and Alaska Native population was estimated at about 2 million. Between the 1980 and the 1990 census, a 38 percent increase occurred in the number of people who identified themselves as American Indians or Alaska Natives. This increase reflects an

About This Chapter: Excerpted from "Diabetes in American Indians and Alaska Natives," a publication of the National Diabetes Information Clearinghouse (NDIC), a service of the National Institute of Diabetes and Digestive and Kidney Diseases (NIDDK), National Institutes of Health (NIH), NIH Publication No. 02-4567, May 2002.

actual rise in the number of people who
identify themselves as part of this
group, as well as improvements in
counting methodology. In 1990, more
than half of the American Indian and
Alaska Native population lived in the
following seven States: Alaska, Arizona, Cali-

fornia, New Mexico, North Carolina, Oklahoma, and Washington. The 1990
census in Alaska showed a total of 85,698 self-identified Alaska Natives.
Alaska Natives include three main population groups: Eskimo, Indian, and
Aleut. Within these three groups are further divisions based on geographic
location and linguistic and cultural differences.

Within the estimated 2 million self-identified American Indians, about
1.2 million live on 33 reservations served by the Indian Health Service (IHS).
Increasingly, tribal organizations are contracting directly with the Federal
Government to operate health care facilities on reservations. The following
data on American Indians are drawn primarily from information about
American Indians living on reservations, not from American Indians living
outside the reservations.

Most American Indians and Alaska Natives with diabetes have type 2
diabetes, which usually develops in adults but can develop in children or
adolescents. Type 2 diabetes is caused by the body's resistance to the action of
insulin and by impaired insulin secretion. It can be managed with healthy eating,
physical activity, oral diabetes medications, and/or injected insulin. Until recently, type 2 diabetes was rarely diagnosed in children and adolescents.
However, type 2 diabetes is now common in American Indian children age
10 and older. A small number of American Indians (about 2 to 4 percent)
have type 1 diabetes, which usually develops before age 20 and is managed
with insulin, healthy eating, and physical activity.

How many American Indians and Alaska Natives have diabetes?

About 15 percent of American Indians and Alaska Natives who receive
care from the Indian Health Service have been diagnosed with diabetes, a
total of 105,000 people. On average, American Indians and Alaska Natives

are 2.6 times as likely to have diagnosed diabetes as non-Hispanic whites of a similar age. The available data probably underestimate the true prevalence of diabetes in this population. For example, 40 to 70 percent of American Indian adults ages 45 to 74 were found to have diabetes in a recent screening study in three geographic areas. Data from the Navajo Health and Nutrition Survey, published in 1997, showed that 22.9 percent of Navajo adults ages 20 and older had diabetes. Fourteen percent had a history of diabetes, but another 7 percent were found to have undiagnosed diabetes during the survey.

Table 8.1. Age-adjusted prevalence of diagnosed diabetes among American Indians/ Alaska Natives, age 20 and older, by group of tribes—United States, 1997.

<u>Group of Tribes</u>	<u>Geographic Area</u>	<u>Prevalence (%)</u>
Alaska	Alaska	4.4
Atlantic	Alabama, Connecticut, Florida, Louisiana, Maine, Mississippi, New York, North Carolina, Pennsylvania, Rhode Island, South Carolina, Tennessee, Texas	21.0
Great Lakes	Michigan, Minnesota, Wisconsin	15.2
Northern Plains	Iowa, Montana, Nebraska, North Dakota, South Dakota, Wyoming	16.3
Pacific Tribes	California, Idaho, Oregon, Washington	7.0
Southern Plains	Kansas, Oklahoma	9.6
Southwest	Arizona, Colorado, Nevada, New Mexico, Utah	13.9

Note: Age-adjusted to the 1980 U.S. population; prevalence is per 100 persons. Data on American Indians/Alaska Natives are from the 1997 Indian Health Service (IHS) Patient Care Component file; excludes data from 27 (representing 12 percent of the population served by IHS) of the 145 IHS service units that report data to the IHS because the data were incomplete.

Source of data: Rios Burrows (1999, July 26).

Type 2 diabetes is becoming increasingly common in youth. Researchers studying 5,274 Pima Indian children from 1967 to 1996 found that the prevalence of type 2 diabetes in girls ages 10 to 14 increased from 0.72 percent in the period 1967 to 1976 to 2.88 percent in the period 1987 to 1996. Reports include an increasing incidence in First Nation populations in Canada.

In 1998, about 70,000 of the 2.3 million self-identified American Indians/ Alaska Natives who receive care from the IHS had diabetes. Diabetes rates for American Indians vary by tribal group, as shown in Table 8.1.

Diabetes is particularly common among middle age and older American Indians and Alaska Natives.

In Pima Indians, the most widely studied American Indian group, the prevalence of type 2 diabetes was approximately 50 percent in individuals ages 30 to 64.

During the period from 1986 to 1993, the prevalence of diabetes in Alaska Natives for all ages (adjusted to the 1980 U.S. population) increased by 29 percent, from 15.2 to 19.6 cases per 1,000 people. Of these, most had type 2 diabetes.

The prevalence of type 2 diabetes in Alaska Natives varies by subgroup:

• Eskimo groups (Inupiaq Eskimos in the northern and northwestern coastal areas and Yup'ik Eskimos in the southwestern coastal regions and St. Lawrence Island) had a prevalence of 12.1 per 1,000 in 1993.

• Indian groups (Athabascan in the interior region; Tlingit, Haida, and Tsimshian in the coastal areas) had a prevalence of 24.3 per 1,000 in 1993.

• Aleut groups (residents of the Aleutian Islands, the Pribilof Islands, the western tip of the Alaska Peninsula, the Kodiak area, and the south-central coastal areas) had a prevalence of 32.6 per 1,000 in 1993.

♣ **It's A Fact!!**
Type 1 diabetes is relatively rare in American Indians and Alaska Natives. Most cases of type 1 diabetes are seen in people who have both American Indian and Caucasian heritage.

What risk factors increase the chance that American Indians and Alaska natives will develop type 2 diabetes?

Two categories of risk factors increase the chance of type 2 diabetes. The first is genetics. The second is medical and lifestyle risk factors, including obesity, diet, and physical inactivity. Individuals with impaired glucose tolerance, impaired fasting glucose, or insulin resistance are at higher risk of progressing to diabetes.

Genetic Risk Factors: Genetic background is a determining factor in the prevalence of type 2 diabetes. In both the Choctaw Indians and the Pima Indians, the more full-blooded individuals were found to have the highest prevalence of type 2 diabetes, as compared with those of more mixed heritage. In Pima Indians, diabetes rates were found to be highest in children whose parents developed diabetes at an early age.

Although the specific genes responsible for the inheritance of type 2 diabetes have not been located, NIDDK scientists studying the Pima Indians have identified a gene called FABP2 that may play a role in insulin resistance. More recent studies have shown that a variant in the PPPIR3 gene that is more common in Pimas than Caucasians is associated with type 2 diabetes and insulin resistance.

Obesity: Obesity is a major risk factor for type 2 diabetes among all races and ethnic groups. Increasing rates of obesity have been measured in many American Indian and Alaska Native communities. In Pima Indians, 95 percent of those with diabetes are overweight.

The study of obesity and energy metabolism in Pima Indians has not identified exact causes but has revealed that Pima Indian families share the trait of a low metabolic rate. This trait is considered predictive of weight gain and development of type 2 diabetes. A "thrifty gene" is also thought to cause a genetic predisposition to obesity, although this gene has not been identified. The thrifty gene theory, first proposed in 1962, suggests that populations of indigenous people who experienced alternating periods of feast and famine gradually adapted by developing a way to store fat more efficiently during periods of plenty to better survive famines.

The degree to which obesity is a risk factor for diabetes depends greatly on the location of the excess weight. Central or upper-body obesity is a stronger risk factor for type 2 diabetes than excess weight carried below the waist. In young Pima Indians, waist-to-hip ratio, a measure of central obesity, was more strongly associated with diabetes than body mass index, a measure of overall obesity.

Diet And Physical Inactivity: Both diet and physical activity have changed for many members of American Indian and Alaska Native groups over the past several decades. Diets are higher in fat and calories than traditional diets; physical activity has decreased. Changes in diet and physical activity are associated with the increased prevalence of type 2 diabetes. For example, Pima Indians living in Mexico who consumed a more traditional diet (less animal fat and more complex carbohydrates) had a lower prevalence of type 2 diabetes than Pima Indians living in Arizona. Pima Indians in Mexico also expended more calories through activity.

Pre-Diabetes (Impaired Glucose Tolerance And Impaired Fasting Glucose): Recent recommendations describe two categories of the physiological state between normal blood glucose and the diabetic range of blood glucose. Individuals are described as having impaired glucose tolerance (a 2-hour glucose value of between 140 and 199 mg/dL during the oral glucose tolerance test) or impaired fasting glucose (a fasting plasma glucose value between 110 and 125 mg/dL).

American Indians with impaired glucose tolerance have a higher incidence of diabetes than those whose glucose tolerance test results are in the normal range.

Hyperinsulinemia And Insulin Resistance: Hyperinsulinemia (higher than normal levels of fasting insulin) and insulin resistance (the inability of the body to use its own insulin to properly control blood glucose) are both associated with an increased risk of developing type 2 diabetes. Hyper-insulinemia often predates diabetes by several years. Studies of Pima Indians have shown that both increased insulin secretion and insulin resistance occur in conjunction with impaired glucose tolerance.

How does diabetes affect American Indian and Alaska native women during pregnancy?

Both long- and short-term consequences of diabetes during pregnancy are evident in American Indians and Alaska Natives. Congenital abnormalities in infants born to women with type 2 diabetes are as common as those observed in women with type 1 diabetes. Other complications seen in pregnancies in women with type 2 diabetes included increased rates of toxemia and perinatal mortality.

Gestational diabetes, in which blood glucose levels are elevated above normal during pregnancy, occurs in about 2 to 5 percent of all American pregnant women. Perinatal problems such as macrosomia (large body size) and neonatal hypoglycemia (low blood sugar) are higher in babies born to women with gestational diabetes. Although blood glucose levels generally return to normal after childbirth, an increased risk of developing gestational diabetes in future pregnancies remains. In addition, studies show that many women with gestational diabetes will develop type 2 diabetes later in life.

The prevalence of gestational diabetes in certain groups of American Indians and Alaska Natives is as follows:

- 14.5 percent of pregnancies in Zuni Indians
- 3.4 percent of deliveries in Navajo Indians
- 5.8 percent of deliveries in Yup'ik Eskimos

Followup studies of American Indian women with gestational diabetes found a high risk of developing subsequent diabetes: 27.5 percent of Pima Indian women developed diabetes within 4 to 8 years, and 30 percent of Zuni Indian women developed diabetes within 6 months to 9 years after pregnancy.

Longitudinal studies of diabetes in Pima Indians have shown that adult offspring of women with diabetes during pregnancy have significantly higher rates of diabetes than adult offspring of women without diabetes, showing the possible effect of the diabetic intrauterine environment. In fact, 45 percent of adult offspring of Pima Indian women who were diagnosed with type 2 diabetes predating pregnancy developed diabetes by age 20 to 24. In comparison, only 1.4 percent of adult offspring of women without diabetes during pregnancy went on to develop diabetes by age 24. The strongest single risk factor for diabetes in Pima children was exposure to diabetes in utero.

How does diabetes affect cardiovascular health in American Indians and Alaska natives?

Ischemic Heart Disease: Diabetes is a major risk factor for cardiovascular disease in all American Indian populations, and cardiovascular disease is the leading cause of death. All heart-related deaths from 1975 to 1984 in Pima Indians occurred in those with diabetes. Recent studies of cardiovascular mortality in Arizona, Oklahoma, North Dakota, and South Dakota revealed that cardiovascular mortality was higher in American Indians compared with that of non-Hispanic whites in the United States.

✎ What's It Mean?

Cerebrovascular: Disease of the blood vessels in the brain. [1]

Intrauterine: Within the uterus. [2]

Ischemia: Decrease in the blood supply to an organ, tissue, or other part caused by the narrowing or blockage of the blood vessels. [1]

Neonatal: Affecting the newborn and especially the human infant during the first month after birth. [3]

Perinatal: Events that occur at or around the time of birth. [4]

Pneumonia: Inflammation of the lungs. Causes of pneumonia include bacteria and viruses. [1]

Toxemia: It is a condition that can occur in a woman in the second half of her pregnancy that can cause serious problems for both her and the baby. It causes high blood pressure, protein in the urine, blood changes and other problems. [1]

Tuberculosis: A bacterial infection caused by Mycobacterium tuberculosis. TB bacteria are spread by airborne droplets expelled from the lungs when a person with active TB coughs, sneezes, or speaks. Exposure to these droplets can lead to infection in the air sacs of the lungs. The immune defenses of healthy people usually prevent TB infection from spreading beyond a very small area of the lungs. [4]

Utero: In the uterus. [2]

Source: [1] "NWHIC Web Site Glossary," U.S. Department of Health and Human Services, Office on Women's Health, cited July 2005; available at http://www.4woman.gov/Glossary. [2] Editor. [3] "Genetics Home Reference Glossary," a service of the U.S. National Library of Medicine, July 2005; available at http://www.ghr.nlm.nih.gov. [4] "HIV Glossary," AIDS info, a service of the U.S. Department of Health and Human Services, September 2002; available at http://www.aidsinfo.nih.gov/ed%5Fresources/glossary.

Stroke: Little information is available on stroke rates in American Indians. The incidence of stroke in Alaska Natives was greatest among Eskimos, followed by Aleuts and Indians. The overall incidence of stroke in Eskimo women was higher than in any other group studied.

Hypertension: Hypertension (high blood pressure) in American Indians in the United States appears to be less prevalent than in the general population. However, recent studies of American Indians in Arizona and Oklahoma showed that the prevalence of hypertension was higher than that of non-Hispanic whites in a national survey.

How do diabetes complications affect American Indians and Alaska natives?

Diabetic Retinopathy: Diabetic retinopathy is a deterioration of the blood vessels in the eye caused by high blood glucose levels. It can lead to impaired vision and, ultimately, to blindness. One study showed a 49 percent prevalence of diabetic retinopathy in Oklahoma Indians. Pima Indians also have excessive rates of diabetic retinopathy.

Cataracts: The incidence of cataract extraction among Pima Indians with diabetes was more than twice the rate of people without diabetes.

Diabetic Nephropathy: From 1987 to 1990, American Indians with diabetes experienced end-stage renal disease (the final stage of kidney disease associated with kidney failure and dialysis) six times more frequently than did non-Hispanic whites. Especially high rates of diabetic nephropathy (kidney disease) were seen in Alaska Native, Cherokee, Chippewa, Navajo, Oklahoma, Pima, Sioux, and Zuni tribes. In 1989, end-stage renal disease was a leading cause of death among Pima Indians with diabetes.

Among Alaska Natives, women were more likely to develop end-stage renal disease and more likely to die of renal failure than men. The overall incidence of dialysis caused by diabetic renal disease from 1986 until 1993 in Alaska Natives was two per 1,000 person-years of diabetes.

Lower Extremity Amputation: Rates of lower extremity amputation are high in some American Indians but vary by tribe. Several studies indicate a higher amputation rate among men than among women. Loss of protective sensation as detected by a screening monofilament test identified diabetic individuals at high risk for amputation and foot ulceration.

Periodontal Disease: Among Pima Indians, the periodontal disease rate was 2.6 times higher in people with diabetes than in those without it. Poor glycemic control among American Indians has been associated with an increased risk of periodontal disease.

Infections: Infections related to diabetes in American Indians are of particular concern. A study in Sioux Indians showed that those with diabetes were 4.4 times more likely to develop tuberculosis than were Sioux Indians without diabetes. Mortality in Pima Indians with infectious diseases is significant, according to a study that found that five out of six people who died from a serious infection (coccidioidomycosis) had diabetes. In 1987, tuberculosis mortality among American Indians was 5.8 times higher than the rate among all races in the United States.

Does diabetes cause an inordinate number of deaths?

From 1984 to 1986, diabetes was the sixth leading cause of death among American Indians and Alaska Natives in the United States.

Because mortality rates are based on the underlying cause of death on death certificates, the impact of diabetes on mortality among American Indians and Alaska Natives has been underestimated. Diabetes contributes to several of the leading causes of death in American Indians: heart disease, cerebrovascular disease, pneumonia, and influenza. In addition, one study found that American Indian heritage was underreported on death certificates by 65 percent. Between 1986 and 1988, the adjusted mortality rate for diabetes in American Indians was 4.3 times the rate in non-Hispanic whites. Age- and sex-adjusted death rate studies of Pima Indians from 1975 to 1984 found that the mortality rate for diabetes was nearly 12 times greater than the 1980 mortality rate for all races in the United States. Both the duration of the disease and the presence of proteinuria (indicating kidney disease) were factors associated with increased mortality.

According to the Alaska Area Native Health Service, the mortality rate for diabetes in Alaska Natives from 1986 to 1993 was 43.2 per 1,000 person-years of diabetes. Average age at death was 70.3 years. Mortality rates were similar for Aleuts, Eskimos, and Indians.

Chapter 9

Genetics And Diabetes

What's Your Risk?

A school nurse anxiously wants to know if there is a reason why several children from her small grade school have been diagnosed with type 1 (juvenile onset) diabetes. Is it an epidemic? Will there be more cases? Is a recent chicken pox outbreak to blame?

A man in his 50s develops type 2 diabetes. His mother developed diabetes in her 60s. Should this man's brother and sister be concerned, too? What about his children's chances of developing diabetes?

A married couple wants to have children, but they are concerned because the husband has type 1 diabetes. They wonder what the risk is that their child would have diabetes.

A couple has three young children. One of the children develops type 1 diabetes. There's no history of diabetes anywhere in either parent's families.

About This Chapter: This chapter begins with "What's Your Risk?" Copyright © 2005 by Joslin Diabetes Center. All rights reserved. Reprinted with permission from The Joslin Diabetes Center website, http://www.joslin.org. Text under the heading "Pima Indians and Diabetes" is from "The Pima Indians, Pathfinders for Health, The Pima Indians and Genetic Research," a publication of the National Diabetes Information Clearinghouse (NDIC), a service of the National Institute of Diabetes and Digestive and Kidney Diseases (NIDDK), National Institutes of Health (NIH), May 2002.

Is this just a fluke? What are the chances the other children will develop diabetes?

Chances are if you or a loved one have diabetes, you may wonder if you inherited it from a family member or you may be concerned that you will pass the disease on to your children.

Researchers at Joslin Diabetes Center report that, while much has been learned about what genetic factors make one more susceptible to developing diabetes than another, many questions remain to be answered. While some people are more likely to get diabetes than others, and in some ways type 2 (adult onset diabetes) is simpler to track than type 1 (juvenile onset) diabetes, the pattern is not always clear.

For more than 20 years researchers in the Epidemiology and Genetics Section at Joslin in Boston (Section Head Andrzej S. Krolewski, M.D., Ph.D., Senior Investigator James H. Warram, M.D., Sc.D., and colleagues) have been studying diabetes incidence and hereditary factors. They are continuing a scientific journey begun by Elliott P. Joslin, M.D., who in 1946 launched a 20-year study to determine the prevalence of diabetes cases in his small hometown of Oxford, MA. Over the years, Joslin researchers have studied many generations of families to determine how best to predict who is at risk for diabetes.

Diabetes affects an estimated 18.2 million Americans (about 5.2 million are undiagnosed and therefore unaware that they have the disease), with an estimated 1.3 million Americans diagnosed each year. Type 2 diabetes

♣ **It's A Fact!!**

According to the American Diabetes Association, type 1 diabetes accounts for 5 to 10 percent of all diagnosed cases of diabetes. Each year, over 13,000 new cases of type 1 diabetes are diagnosed in children and teenagers, making it one of the most common chronic diseases in American children.

Source: Copyright © 2005 by Joslin Diabetes Center. All rights reserved.

represents about 90 to 95 percent of the cases and is more common in people in their 40s and beyond, in certain ethnic groups, and in those who are obese and sedentary.

People with type 1 diabetes do not produce insulin, a hormone that regulates how cells obtain energy from food; in type 2, the pancreas produces too little insulin or the body is not able to properly use insulin the body does produce. Diabetes is a major cause of heart disease, blindness, kidney disease, nerve damage, and other complications.

According to Dr. Warram, several factors are central to the risk question: the person with diabetes has most likely inherited a predisposition to the disease, and secondly, something in the environment triggers the disease. For the average American, the chance of developing type 1 diabetes by age 70 years is 1 in 100 (1 percent), while the corresponding chances of getting type 2 diabetes are at 1 in 9 (11 percent). Knowing what the odds are is one thing; but one can still get the disease even if he or she is not at apparent high risk.

Type 1 Diabetes Odds

Just who is at risk for developing type 1 diabetes? Here's a sampling of what Dr. Warram, a Lecturer in Epidemiology at Harvard School of Public Health, said is known:

- If an immediate relative (parent, brother, sister, son, or daughter) has type 1 diabetes, one's risk of developing type 1 diabetes is 10 to 20 times the risk of the general population. Your risk can go from 1 in 100 to roughly 1 in 10 or possibly higher, depending on which family member has the diabetes and when they developed it.

- If one child in a family has type 1 diabetes, their siblings have about a 1 in 10 risk of developing it by age 50.

- The risk for a child of a parent with type 1 diabetes is lower if it is the mother, rather than the father, who has diabetes. "If the father has it, the risk is about 1 in 10 (10 percent) that his child will develop type 1 diabetes—the same as the risk to a sibling of an affected child," Dr. Warram says. On the other hand, if the mother has type 1 diabetes and is age 25 or younger when the child is born, the risk is reduced to 1 in 25 (4 percent). If the mother is over age 25, the risk drops to 1 in 100—virtually the same as the average American.

- If one of the parents developed type 1 diabetes before age 11, their child's risk of developing type 1 diabetes is somewhat higher than these figures and lower if the parent was diagnosed after their 11th birthday.

- About 1 in 7 people with type 1 has a condition known as type 2 polyglandular autoimmune syndrome. In addition to type 1 diabetes, these people have thyroid disease, malfunctioning adrenal glands, and sometimes other immune disorders. For those with this syndrome, the child's risk of having the syndrome, including type 1 diabetes, is 1 in 2, according to the American Diabetes Association (ADA).

Caucasians (whites) have a higher risk of type 1 diabetes than any other race. Whether this is due to differences in environment or genes is unclear. Even among whites, most people who are susceptible do not develop diabetes. Therefore, scientists are studying what environmental factors may be at work. Genes influencing the function of the immune system are the most closely linked to type 1 diabetes susceptibility, regardless of race. One of those genes is HLA-DR. Most Caucasians with diabetes carry alleles (gene variants) 3 and/or 4 of the HLA-DR gene. The HLA-DR7 allele plays a role in diabetes in blacks, while HLA-DR9 allele is important in diabetes among Japanese.

Climate And Clusters

Among Caucasians, diabetes risk varies geographically. In general, the risk is higher in Northern Europeans than Southern Europeans. While climate may contribute to this, the fact that Sardinia in the Mediterranean also has a high risk goes against this theory. Generally the number of new cases over time fluctuates up and down, making it difficult to find an overall pattern. In recent decades, there has been an increase in type 1 diabetes in the United States and Europe. While Asians generally have a much lower incidence of type 1 diabetes, Japan is also experiencing an increasing incidence. "The gene pool doesn't change much within one generation, so there must be an environmental or behavioral factor involved," Dr. Warram says.

Temporal clusters of type 1 diabetes cases (i.e. those that occur around the same time, whether within families, a school or a geographical region), prompt people to suspect an environmental agent. However, no consistent explanation has come up for these clusters, and it is impossible to rule out the possibility of just coincidence. Given the fact that the development of diabetes takes many years in most cases, a clustering in time seems more likely due to chance than a common cause, Dr. Warram says. "From what we know, the autoimmune process leading to the destruction of insulin-producing beta cells in the pancreas is quite long. People can have antibodies signaling damage to the beta cells for many years without developing diabetes," Dr. Warram says.

Take the "outbreak" at the grade school mentioned above. Chances are, the youngsters were not attending the same school or even living in the same neighborhood when the lengthy autoimmune process leading to diabetes began. (In that process, the body's disease-fighting immune system mal-functions, turning against the body's own tissues and destroying them.) While we can't be certain, it seems unlikely that we could observe a particular expo-sure that caused the youngsters to develop diabetes at the same time," Dr. Warram says. "Most likely it's a matter of chance. While it is not comforting to say rare events can happen by chance, rare events are happening all the time within a given population, and the chances of them occurring in one place, like a school, is high."

Trauma As A Trigger

Some people have questioned whether a body trauma, like a car crash, or a viral infection like mumps, could trigger the onset of type 1 diabetes. Such events increase the body's insulin requirement and strain the insulin produc-tion system if it is being destroyed by a malfunctioning immune system. "As the demands on the body increase, it can tip the body's insulin production system over the edge," Dr. Warram says. But the trauma itself did not cause the diabetes, he says.

Much has been said about a possible link between Coxsackie virus, which causes human diseases such as meningitis, and the triggering of type 1 dia-betes. "You can't dismiss the fact that sometimes the virus has been present, but its connection with the diabetes is unclear," Dr. Warram says. Scientists do have some significant evidence that mumps does not trigger diabetes, however. A Maryland study showed that despite a great decline in mumps cases after the mumps vaccine was introduced 30 years ago, the incidence of type 1 diabetes did not change.

Some scientists believe early diet may have a role. Prolonged breast-feeding is less common in children who developed type 1 diabetes. While some studies have pointed to exposure to cow's milk, Dr. Warram says much remains to be learned before we can assess the importance of this mechanism. To be prudent, mothers of infants at high risk of developing diabetes may want to breast-feed as long as possible and rely on cow's milk only in moderation after the baby is weaned.

Tracking Type 2 Diabetes

Patients with type 2 diabetes are more likely to know of a relative with diabetes than patients with type 1 and, therefore, suppose that diabetes "runs in the family." To some extent the appearance of "clustering" of type 2 diabetes in families is simply the consequence of the fact that type 2 is so much more common than type 1 diabetes in the general population. Moreover, the occurrence of multiple cases in a family may reflect shared "environmental risk factors," such as obesity and sedentary lifestyle, and does not imply necessarily the sharing of a diabetes gene. In general, the risk of diabetes for a sibling of a patient with type 2 diabetes is about the same as that in the general population. However, there are some exceptions to this general statement. If the patient developed diabetes despite being lean, then the sibling's risk is about twice the general population risk. Or, if the patient has a parent with type 2 diabetes, the sibling's risk is almost three times the general population risk. If both parents have type 2 diabetes, the sibling has a fourfold risk, or nearly a 50% chance of developing diabetes.

The genetics of type 2 diabetes is complex. While type 2 diabetes may have a strong genetic basis in some patients (something less than a third of them), the development of diabetes in most patients is dependent upon the effects of environmental and behavioral factors (obesity and sedentary lifestyle) on an underlying susceptibility that is poorly understood.

What About MODY?

Over Dr. Warram's desk is a chart of several generations of one family. About half of the people in the family have developed a form of type 2 diabetes called MODY (maturity-onset diabetes of the young) that typically develops in people in their teens and 20s. The family is one of about 50 families with MODY studied by the Joslin researchers. "In this family, every generation is affected, and every family member with MODY had a parent with MODY," Dr. Warram says.

Joslin researchers and others have identified about six genes that produce MODY, but they only account for the diabetes in about one-third of the families. "The diabetes in the rest of the families so far is unexplained," he says.

Similar patterns can be found in studies of families with the more common form of type 2 diabetes, only the age of onset differs.

The susceptibility to certain diabetes complications also seems to be linked in some ways with genetics. For patients with susceptibility genes for complications, good blood glucose control is still an important mitigating factor.

Scientists at Joslin and elsewhere are studying genetic factors that may make some people with diabetes more susceptible to complications as well.

An Individual Decision

If there's one thing Dr. Warram feels strongly about, it's not to advise people considering having a baby or marrying someone with diabetes in the family. "I do not mind telling people what we know about diabetes risks, but I am not qualified to give an opinion about their choice. These are matters of personal choice and what's important to me may not be important to someone else," he says.

"To be told a child has a 4 percent or 10 percent risk of diabetes sounds very absolute and scientific," he says. "But a myriad of other things can go wrong with a child, medically and socially, and these risks cannot be measured precisely. Also, there are a myriad of other things that can go right for a child. Even if a child does develop diabetes, it needn't prevent him or her from finding success and happiness in life. "Raising children, whether they are your own or adopted, is an experience involving risks of great rewards and risks of great costs that can't really be known in advance. If a number can be attached to one of those risks, should it weigh more than the others?"

Pima Indians And Diabetes

Why do so many Pima Indians have diabetes? The question is simple, but the answers are not. They are part of a very complex puzzle that National

> ### ♣ It's A Fact!!
> ### What are the different ways
> ### in which a genetic condition can be inherited?
>
> Some genetic conditions are caused by mutations in a single gene. These conditions are usually inherited in one of several straightforward patterns, depending on the gene involved.
>
> **Autosomal Dominant.** One mutated copy of the gene in each cell is sufficient for a person to be affected by an autosomal dominant disorder. Each affected person usually has one affected parent. Autosomal dominant disorders tend to occur in every generation of an affected family.
>
> **Autosomal Recessive.** Two mutated copies of the gene are present in each cell when a person has an autosomal recessive disorder. An affected person usually has unaffected parents who each carry a single copy of the mutated gene (and are referred to as carriers). Autosomal recessive disorders are typically not seen in every generation of an affected family.
>
> **X-Linked Dominant.** X-linked dominant disorders are caused by mutations in genes on the X chromosome. Females are more frequently affected than males, and the chance of passing on an X-linked dominant disorder differs between men and women. Families with an X-linked dominant disorder often have both affected males and affected females in each generation. A striking characteristic of X-linked inheritance is that fathers cannot pass X-linked traits to their sons (no male-to-male transmission).

Institutes of Health (NIH) researchers are trying to decode through genetic research.

There are approximately 100,000 genes packed into 23 pairs of chromosomes in each person. Within a gene, chemicals form individual codes, like words, which tell the cells of the body what to do. It is the code within a gene that directs the body to grow skin, and determines whether the skin is brown, yellow, black, or white; to form hair and bone; to circulate blood and hormones such as adrenalin and insulin; and to perform every other biological process in the body.

X-Linked Recessive. X-linked recessive disorders are also caused by mutations in genes on the X chromosome. Males are more frequently affected than females, and the chance of passing on the disorder differs between men and women. Families with an X-linked recessive disorder often have affected males, but rarely affected females, in each generation. A striking characteristic of X-linked inheritance is that fathers cannot pass X-linked traits to their sons (no male-to-male transmission).

Mitochondrial. This type of inheritance, also known as maternal inheritance, applies to genes in mitochondrial DNA. Mitochondria, which are structures in each cell that convert molecules into energy, each contain a small amount of DNA. Because only egg cells contribute mitochondria to the developing embryo, only females can pass on mitochondrial conditions to their children. Mitochondrial disorders can appear in every generation of a family and can affect both males and females, but fathers do not pass mitochondrial traits to their children.

Many other disorders are caused by a combination of the effects of multiple genes or by interactions between genes and the environment. Such disorders are more difficult to analyze because their genetic causes are often unclear, and they do not follow the patterns of inheritance described above. Examples of conditions caused by multiple genes or gene/environment interactions include heart disease, diabetes, schizophrenia, and certain types of cancer.

Source: Genetics Home Reference (http://ghr.nlm.nih.gov), a service of the U.S. National Library of Medicine®, National Institutes of Health (NIH), Department of Health and Human Services, May 2005.

♣ It's A Fact!!
If a genetic disorder runs in my family, what are the chances that my children will have the condition?

When a genetic disorder is diagnosed in a family, family members often want to know the likelihood that they or their children will develop the condition. This can be difficult to predict in some cases because many factors influence a person's chances. One important factor is how the condition is inherited. For example:

- A person affected by an autosomal dominant disorder has a 50 percent chance of passing the mutated gene to each child. There is also a 50 percent chance that a child will not inherit the mutated gene.

- For an autosomal recessive disorder, two unaffected people who each carry one copy of the mutated gene (carriers) have a 25 percent chance with each pregnancy of having a child affected by the disorder. There is a 75 percent chance with each pregnancy that a child will be unaffected.

- The chance of passing on an X-linked dominant condition differs between men and women because men have one X chromosome and one Y chromosome, while women have two X chromosomes. A man passes on his Y chromosome to all of his sons and his X chromosome to all of his daughters. Therefore, the sons of a man with an X-linked dominant disorder will not be affected, and his daughters will all inherit the condition. A woman passes on one or the other of her X chromosomes to each child. Therefore, a woman with an X-linked dominant disorder has a 50 percent chance of having an affected daughter or son with each pregnancy.

- Because of the difference in sex chromosomes, the probability of passing on an X-linked recessive disorder also differs between men and women.

Finding the gene or genes that may increase a person's risk for getting diabetes and obesity is the most effective way scientists have to learn what's wrong in a diabetic person.

With the help of the Pima Indians, NIH scientists have already learned that diabetes develops when a person's body doesn't use insulin effectively.

The sons of a man with an X-linked recessive disorder will not be affected, and his daughters will carry one copy of the mutated gene. With each pregnancy, a woman who carries an X-linked recessive disorder has a 50 percent chance of having sons who are affected and a 50 percent chance of having daughters who carry one copy of the mutated gene.

It is important to note that the chance of passing on a genetic condition applies equally to each pregnancy. For example, if a couple has a child with an autosomal recessive disorder, the chance of having another child with the disorder is still 25 percent (or 1 in 4). Having one child with a disorder does not protect future children from inheriting the condition. Conversely, having a child without the condition does not mean that future children will definitely be affected.

Although the chances of inheriting a genetic condition appear straightforward, in some cases factors such as a person's family history and the results of genetic testing can modify those chances. In addition, some people with a disease-causing mutation never develop any health problems or may experience only mild symptoms of the disorder. If a disease that runs in a family does not have a clear-cut inheritance pattern, predicting the likelihood that a person will develop the condition can be particularly difficult.

Because estimating the chance of developing or passing on a genetic disorder can be complex, genetics professionals can help people understand these chances and make informed decisions about their health.

Source: Genetics Home Reference (http://ghr.nlm.nih.gov), a service of the U.S. National Library of Medicine ®, National Institutes of Health (NIH), Department of Health and Human Services, May 2005.

They know that other genes probably influence some people's bodies to burn energy at a slow rate, and/or to want to eat more, making it more likely that they will become overweight. Being overweight, in turn, puts a person at even higher risk for diabetes. Because they have learned this over 30 years of working with the Pima Indians, NIH scientists now are able to test ways to prevent the disease with low-fat diets and regular exercise.

When scientists find the codes for the genes that contribute to diabetes and obesity, they will be able to study how the genes work, and how the changes that result might contribute to disease. Then they will have the best clues available to design treatments and cures.

DNA, each human being's personal collection of genes, is as individual as a thumbprint. Because the code for a particular gene can be slightly different in each person, tracking genes is difficult, time-consuming work. It is possible to do this work only when scientists have the cooperation of large families.

Mormon families in Salt Lake City helped researchers find a gene for colon cancer, and a large group of related families in Venezuela contributed their blood and skin samples so researchers could identify the gene for Huntington's disease. Now Pima families from the Gila River Indian Community are making it possible for the National Institute of Diabetes and Digestive and Kidney Diseases (NIDDK) researchers to search for diabetes and obesity genes.

If it were not for families of Pima Indian volunteers and technology developed in the last 10 years, it would not be possible to search for the genetic causes of so complex a disease as diabetes, according to Dr. Clifton Bogardus of NIDDK.

"We got into this work because of Pima families," Dr. Bogardus says. "NIDDK scientists, including Drs. Bennett, Knowler, and Pettitt, have studied well over 90 percent of the people on the reservation at least once. We know the families, and DNA has been collected from them routinely since the mid 1980s."

Shortly after that, other scientists began to develop ways of creating maps that show where genes are located on chromosomes in cells. They learned how to cut a fragment of DNA, and find its code. Because fragments of DNA will naturally attach to complementary fragments like a zipper, scientists learned how to identify unfamiliar pieces of DNA by using familiar fragments that were electronically labeled. If the labeled DNA found a match, scientists were able to use x-ray film to make a picture of the unfamiliar DNA fragment.

Remember!!

Some diseases are caused by bacteria or viruses that infect the body and make it sick. Others, such as diabetes, occur because a gene's code causes it to function differently under some circumstances. For instance, if a person has a gene that makes that person likely to get diabetes, eating a lot of high fat food over time may increase that person's chance of getting sick. On the other hand, eating lower fat foods such as fruits and vegetables and exercising each day may help to prevent the disease. A person can't choose his or her genes, but can choose what to eat and whether or not to exercise.

Source: National Institute of Diabetes and Digestive and Kidney Diseases, 2002.

When researchers have volunteers from large families of several generations, whose medical and genetic history is well known to them, blood samples from those volunteers are extremely valuable in learning about a disease. Using laboratory techniques, they can separate the volunteers' DNA from their blood, and compare DNA from family members who have disease and those who do not.

The researchers look for a piece of DNA shared only by members of a family who have disease. When they find the same genetic variation in many people with disease, that variation is called a marker. Because a marker and a gene that helps cause disease are often inherited together, researchers can then use that marker like a signpost to search for the sought-after gene itself.

Beginning in 1983 and continuing for 10 years, NIDDK studied the genetic codes of almost 300 non-diabetic Pima Indians in great detail. "We looked at body composition, how well a person produced insulin, how well that person's cells responded to insulin, and other factors. After a number of years, some of the volunteers developed diabetes, and we were able to determine that insulin resistance and obesity were major predictors of disease," Dr. Bogardus explains.

Because diabetes is such a complex disease, Dr. Bogardus and his staff are attempting to narrow their search by first looking for the genetic causes of physical conditions that can lead to diabetes, such as the genes that influence a person's cells to secrete less and respond less to insulin that is needed to regulate blood sugar.

In 1993, they identified a gene called FABP2 that may contribute to insulin resistance. This gene makes an intestinal fatty acid binding protein using one of two amino acids. When the gene makes the protein with threonine, one of those amino acids, the body seems to absorb more fatty acids from the fat in meals. NIH scientists think that could lead to a higher level of certain fats and fatty acids in the blood, which could contribute to insulin resistance.

Another group of NIH scientists, led by Dr. Michael Prochazka and Dr. Bruce Thompson, are developing a genetic map for the Pima Indians, a tool that could be very useful in defining what causes so much diabetes in the community. They have already identified a number of markers different from those in the white population.

Researchers sometimes get unexpected results leading to further work, even when they have carefully thought out a project. While studying how a person's cells respond to insulin, biochemist Dr. David Mott identified an enzyme called protein phosphatase 1 that seems to play a role in insulin resistance. "Now it turns out there are actually three of these protein phosphatase enzymes," Dr. Bogardus explains, "so we're trying to figure out which of the three is the most important. We're also trying to find out if there's a difference in one of those three genes in the Pima Indians," he adds.

The NIH gene-seekers hope to answer many questions that could make better health an expectation for diabetes-prone Pima Indians. How do these genes work? What switches these genes on and off? How does a person's lifestyle contribute to disease when these genes are present? Is one gene missing some important chemical? If so, is there a substitute for that chemical's activity?

When they have these answers, doctors may be able to say why the Pima Indians and other non-whites get diabetes so often. They will be better able to identify those who are likely to become diabetic. Most importantly, they will have the pieces of the diabetic puzzle that could be the key to preventing diabetes in new generations of Pima Indians.

Chapter 10

Can Diabetes Be Prevented?

The Diabetes Prevention Program (DPP) was a major clinical trial, or research study, aimed at discovering whether either diet and exercise or the oral diabetes drug metformin (Glucophage) could prevent or delay the onset of type 2 diabetes in people with impaired glucose tolerance (IGT).

The answer is yes. In fact, the DPP found that over the 3 years of the study, diet and exercise sharply reduced the chances that a person with IGT would develop diabetes. Metformin also reduced risk, although less dramatically. The DPP resolved these questions so quickly that, on the advice of an external monitoring board, the program was halted a year early. The researchers published their findings in the February 7, 2002, issue of the *New England Journal of Medicine*.

DPP Study Design And Goals

In the DPP, participants from 27 clinical centers around the country were randomly split into different treatment groups. The first group, called the lifestyle intervention group, received intensive training in diet, exercise, and behavior modification. By eating less fat and fewer calories and exercising

About This Chapter: Excerpted from "Diabetes Prevention Program," a publication of the National Diabetes Information Clearinghouse (NDIC), a service of the National Institute of Diabetes and Digestive and Kidney Diseases (NIDDK), National Institutes of Health (NIH), NIH Publication No. 04-5099, May 2004.

for a total of 150 minutes a week, they aimed to lose 7 percent of their body weight and maintain that loss.

The second group took 850 mg of metformin twice a day. The third group received placebo pills instead of metformin. The metformin and placebo groups also received information on diet and exercise, but no intensive counseling efforts. A fourth group was treated with the drug troglitazone (Rezulin), but this part of the study was discontinued after researchers discovered that troglitazone can cause serious liver damage.

All 3,234 study participants were overweight and had IGT, which are well-recognized risk factors for the development of type 2 diabetes. In addition, 45 percent of the participants were from minority groups—African American, Hispanic American/Latino, Asian American or Pacific Islander, or American Indian—which are at increased risk of developing diabetes.

Type 2 Diabetes And Pre-Diabetes

Diabetes is a disorder that affects the way your body uses digested food for growth and energy. Normally, the food you eat is broken down into glucose. The glucose then passes into your bloodstream, where it is used by your cells for growth and energy. For glucose to reach your cells, however, insulin must be present. Insulin is a hormone produced by your pancreas, a hand-sized gland behind your stomach.

Most people with type 2 diabetes have two problems: the pancreas may not produce enough insulin, and fat, muscle, and liver cells cannot use it effectively. This means that glucose builds up in the blood, overflows into the urine, and passes out of the body—without fulfilling its role as the body's main source of fuel.

About 18.2 million people in the United States have diabetes. Of those, 13 million are diagnosed and 5.2 million are undiagnosed. Ninety to 95 percent of people with diabetes have type 2 diabetes. Diabetes is the main cause of kidney failure, limb amputation, and new-onset blindness in American adults. People with diabetes are also two to four times more likely than people without diabetes to develop heart disease.

Pre-diabetes, also called impaired glucose tolerance (IGT) or impaired fasting glucose (IFG), is a condition in which your blood glucose (blood sugar) levels are higher than normal but not high enough for a diagnosis of diabetes. Having pre-diabetes puts you at higher risk for developing type 2 diabetes. If you have pre-diabetes, you are also at increased risk for developing heart disease.

You are more likely to develop type 2 diabetes if

- you are overweight.

- you are 45 years old or older.

- you have a parent, brother, or sister with diabetes.

- your family background is African American, American Indian, Asian American, Hispanic American/Latino, or Pacific Islander.

- you have had gestational diabetes or gave birth to at least one baby weighing more than 9 pounds.

- your blood pressure is 140/90 or higher, or you have been told that you have high blood pressure.

- your HDL cholesterol is 35 or lower, or your triglyceride level is 250 or higher.

- you are fairly inactive, or you exercise fewer than three times a week.

In a cross-section of U.S. adults aged 40 to 74 tested during the period 1988 to 1994, 33.8 percent had IFG, 15.4 percent had IGT, and 40.1 percent had pre-diabetes (IGT or IFG or both). Applying these percentages to the 2000 U.S. population, about 35 million adults aged 40 to 74 would have IFG, 16 million would have IGT, and 41 million would have pre-diabetes. Those with pre-diabetes are likely to develop type 2 diabetes within 10 years, unless they take steps to prevent or delay diabetes. The results of the Diabetes Prevention Program showed that modest weight loss and regular exercise could prevent or delay type 2 diabetes.

DPP Results

The DPP's striking results tell us that millions of high-risk people can use diet, exercise, and behavior modification to avoid developing type 2 diabetes. The DPP also suggests that metformin is effective in delaying the onset of diabetes.

Participants in the lifestyle intervention group—those receiving intensive counseling on effective diet, exercise, and behavior modification—reduced their risk of developing diabetes by 58 percent. This finding was true across all participating ethnic groups and for both men and women. Lifestyle changes worked particularly well for participants aged 60 and older, reducing their risk by 71 percent. About 5 percent of the lifestyle intervention group developed diabetes each year during the study period, compared with 11 percent in those who did not get the intervention. Researchers think that weight loss—achieved through better eating habits and exercise—reduces the risk of diabetes by improving the ability of the body to use insulin and process glucose.

> **♣ It's A Fact!!**
> Millions of high-risk people can use diet, exercise, and behavior modification to avoid developing type 2 diabetes.

Participants taking metformin reduced their risk of developing diabetes by 31 percent. Metformin was effective for both men and women, but it was least effective in people aged 45 and older. Metformin was most effective in people 25 to 44 years old and in those with a body mass index of 35 or higher (at least 60 pounds overweight). About 7.8 percent of the metformin group developed diabetes each year during the study, compared with 11 percent of the group receiving the placebo.

Chapter 11

How Do Doctors Diagnose Diabetes?

The following tests are used for diagnosis:

• A fasting plasma glucose test measures your blood glucose after you have gone at least 8 hours without eating. This test is used to detect diabetes or pre-diabetes.

• An oral glucose tolerance test measures your blood glucose after you have gone at least 8 hours without eating and 2 hours after you drink a glucose-containing beverage. This test can be used to diagnose diabetes or pre-diabetes.

• In a random plasma glucose test, your doctor checks your blood glucose without regard to when you ate your last meal. This test, along with an assessment of symptoms, is used to diagnose diabetes but not pre-diabetes.

Positive test results should be confirmed by repeating the fasting plasma glucose test or the oral glucose tolerance test on a different day.

About This Chapter: Excerpted from "Diagnosis of Diabetes," a publication of the National Diabetes Information Clearinghouse (NDIC), a service of the National Institute of Diabetes and Digestive and Kidney Diseases (NIDDK), National Institutes of Health (NIH), NIH Publication No. 05-4642, January 2005.

Fasting Plasma Glucose (FPG) Test

The FPG is the preferred test for diagnosing diabetes due to convenience and is most reliable when done in the morning. Results and their meaning are shown in Table 11.1. If your fasting glucose level is 100 to 125 mg/dL, you have a form of pre-diabetes called impaired fasting glucose (IFG), meaning that you are more likely to develop type 2 diabetes but do not have it yet. A level of 126 mg/dL or above, confirmed by repeating the test on another day, means that you have diabetes.

Table 11.1. Fasting Plasma Glucose Test

Plasma Glucose Result (mg/dL)	Diagnosis
99 and below	Normal
100 to 125	Pre-diabetes (impaired fasting glucose)
126 and above	Diabetes*

*Confirmed by repeating the test on a different day.

Oral Glucose Tolerance Test (OGTT)

Research has shown that the OGTT is more sensitive than the FPG test for diagnosing pre-diabetes, but it is less convenient to administer. The OGTT requires you to fast for at least 8 hours before the test. Your plasma glucose is measured immediately before and 2 hours after you drink a liquid containing 75 grams of glucose dissolved in water. Results and what they mean are shown in Table 11.2. If your blood glucose level is between 140 and 199 mg/dL 2 hours after drinking the liquid, you have a form of pre-diabetes called impaired glucose tolerance or IGT, meaning

Table 11.2. Oral Glucose Tolerance Test

2-Hour Plasma Glucose Result (mg/dL)	Diagnosis
139 and below	Normal
140 to 199	Pre-diabetes (impaired glucose tolerance)
200 and above	Diabetes*

*Confirmed by repeating the test on a different day.

Table 11.3. Gestational Diabetes: Above-Normal: Results for the Oral Glucose Tolerance Test

When	Plasma Glucose Result (mg/dL)
Fasting	95 or higher
At 1 hour	180 or higher
At 2 hours	155 or higher
At 3 hours	140 or higher

Note: Some laboratories use other numbers for this test.

that you are more likely to develop type 2 diabetes but do not have it yet. A 2-hour glucose level of 200 mg/dL or above, confirmed by repeating the test on another day, means that you have diabetes.

Gestational diabetes is also diagnosed based on plasma glucose values measured during the OGTT. Blood glucose levels are checked four times during the test. If your blood glucose levels are above normal at least twice during the test, you have gestational diabetes. Table 11.3 shows the above-normal results for the OGTT for gestational diabetes.

Random Plasma Glucose Test

A random blood glucose level of 200 mg/dL or more, plus presence of the following symptoms, can mean that you have diabetes:

• Increased urination

• Increased thirst

• Unexplained weight loss

Other symptoms include fatigue, blurred vision, increased hunger, and sores that do not heal. Your doctor will check your blood glucose level on another day using the FPG or the OGTT to confirm the diagnosis.

Chapter 12

Diabetes Statistics

Total Prevalence Of Diabetes In The United States, All Ages, 2002

- **Total:** 18.2 million people—6.3 percent of the population—have diabetes:
    - **Diagnosed:** 13 million people
    - **Undiagnosed:** 5.2 million people

Prevalence Of Diagnosed Diabetes Among People Under 20 Years Of Age, United States, 2002

- About 210,000 people under 20 years of age have diabetes. This represents 0.26 percent of all people in this age group.

Although type 2 diabetes is a problem among youth, nationally representative data to monitor diabetes trends among youth are not available. Clinic-based reports and regional studies indicate that type 2 diabetes is becoming more common among children and adolescents, particularly in American Indians, African Americans, and Hispanic/Latinos.

About This Chapter: Excerpted from "National Diabetes Statistics," a publication of the National Diabetes Information Clearinghouse (NDIC), a service of the National Institute of Diabetes and Digestive and Kidney Diseases (NIDDK), National Institutes of Health (NIH), NIH Publication No. 05-3892, December 2004.

Total Prevalence Of Diabetes Among People Aged 20 Years Or Older, United States, 2002

- **Age 20 years or older:** 18 million; 8.7 percent of all people in this age group have diabetes.

- **Age 60 years or older:** 8.6 million; 18.3 percent of all people in this age group have diabetes.

> **♣ It's A Fact!!**
> Approximately one in every 400 to 500 children and adolescents has type 1 diabetes.

- **Men:** 8.7 million; 8.7 percent of all men aged 20 years or older have diabetes.

- **Women:** 9.3 million; 8.7 percent of all women aged 20 years or older have diabetes.

Total Prevalence Of Diabetes By Race/Ethnicity Among People Aged 20 Years Or Older, United States, 2002

- **Non-Hispanic whites:** 12.5 million; 8.4 percent of all non-Hispanic whites aged 20 years or older have diabetes.

- **Non-Hispanic blacks:** 2.7 million; 11.4 percent of all non-Hispanic blacks aged 20 years or older have diabetes. On average, non-Hispanic blacks are 1.6 times as likely to have diabetes as non-Hispanic whites of similar age.

- **Hispanic/Latino Americans:** 2.0 million; 8.2 percent of all Hispanic/Latino Americans aged 20 years or older have diabetes. On average, Hispanic/Latino Americans are 1.5 times more likely to have diabetes than non-Hispanic whites of similar age. Mexican Americans, the largest Hispanic/Latino subgroup, are over twice as likely to have diabetes as non-Hispanic whites of similar age. Similarly, residents of Puerto Rico are 1.8 times more likely to have diagnosed diabetes than U.S. non-Hispanic whites. Sufficient data are not available to derive more specific current estimates for other Hispanic/Latino groups.

- **American Indians and Alaska Natives who receive care from the Indian Health Service (IHS):** 110,814; 14.9 percent of American Indians and Alaska Natives aged 20 years or older and receiving care from IHS have diabetes. At the regional level, diabetes is least common among Alaska Natives (8.2 percent) and most common among American Indians in the Southeastern United States (27.8 percent) and southern Arizona (27.8 percent). On average, American Indians and Alaska Natives are 2.2 times as likely to have diabetes as non-Hispanic whites of similar age.

- **Asian Americans and Native Hawaiian or other Pacific Islanders:** In 2002, Native Hawaiians and Japanese and Filipino residents of Hawaii aged 20 years or older were approximately two times as likely to have diagnosed diabetes as white residents of Hawaii of similar age. Prevalence data for diabetes among other Pacific Islanders or Asian Americans are limited, but some groups within these populations are at increased risk for diabetes.

Incidence Of Diabetes, United States, 2002

- New cases diagnosed per year: 1.3 million people aged 20 years or older.

Deaths Among People With Diabetes, United States, 2000

- Diabetes was the sixth leading cause of death listed on U.S. death certificates in 2000. This ranking is based on the 69,301 death certificates in which diabetes was listed as the underlying cause of death. Altogether, diabetes contributed to 213,062 deaths.

- Diabetes is likely to be underreported as a cause of death. Studies have found that only about 35 percent to 40 percent of decedents with diabetes have diabetes listed anywhere on the death certificate and only about 10 percent to 15 percent have it listed as the underlying cause of death.

- Overall, the risk for death among people with diabetes is about two times that of people without diabetes.

Complications Of Diabetes In The United States

Heart Disease And Stroke

- Heart disease is the leading cause of diabetes-related deaths. Adults with diabetes have heart disease death rates about two to four times higher than adults without diabetes.

- The risk for stroke is two to four times higher among people with diabetes.

- About 65 percent of deaths among people with diabetes are due to heart disease and stroke.

High Blood Pressure

- About 73 percent of adults with diabetes have blood pressure greater than or equal to 130/80 mm Hg or use prescription medications for hypertension.

Blindness

- Diabetes is the leading cause of new cases of blindness among adults aged 20 to 74 years.

- Diabetic retinopathy causes 12,000 to 24,000 new cases of blindness each year.

Kidney Disease

- Diabetes is the leading cause of end-stage renal disease, accounting for 44 percent of new cases.

- In 2001, 42,813 people with diabetes began treatment for end-stage renal disease.

- In 2001, a total of 142,963 people with end-stage renal disease due to diabetes were living on chronic dialysis or with a kidney transplant.

Nervous System Disease

- About 60 percent to 70 percent of people with diabetes have mild to severe forms of nervous system damage. The results of such damage include impaired sensation or pain in the feet or hands, slowed digestion of food in the stomach, carpal tunnel syndrome, and other nerve problems.

- Severe forms of diabetic nerve disease are a major contributing cause of lower-extremity amputations.

Amputations

- More than 60 percent of nontraumatic lower-limb amputations occur among people with diabetes.

- In 2000–2001, about 82,000 nontraumatic lower-limb amputations were performed annually among people with diabetes.

Dental Disease

- Periodontal (gum) disease is more common among people with diabetes. Among young adults, those with diabetes have about twice the risk of those without diabetes.

- Almost one-third of people with diabetes have severe periodontal diseases with loss of attachment of the gums to the teeth measuring 5 millimeters or more.

Complications Of Pregnancy

- Poorly controlled diabetes before conception and during the first trimester of pregnancy can cause major birth defects in 5 percent to 10 percent of pregnancies and spontaneous abortions in 15 percent to 20 percent of pregnancies.

- Poorly controlled diabetes during the second and third trimesters of pregnancy can result in excessively large babies, posing a risk to the mother and the child.

Other Complications

- Uncontrolled diabetes often leads to biochemical imbalances that can cause acute life-threatening events, such as diabetic ketoacidosis and hyperosmolar (nonketotic) coma.

• People with diabetes are more susceptible to many other illnesses and, once they acquire these illnesses, often have worse prognoses. For example, they are more likely to die with pneumonia or influenza than people who do not have diabetes.

Cost Of Diabetes In The United States, 2002

• **Total (direct and indirect):** $132 billion

  • **Direct medical costs:** $92 billion

✎ What's It Mean?

Blood Pressure: The force of the blood against the artery walls. Two levels of blood pressure are measured: the highest, or systolic, occurs when the heart pumps blood into the blood vessels, and the lowest, or diastolic, occurs when the heart rests. [1]

Carpal Tunnel Syndrome: The name for a group of problems that includes swelling, pain, tingling, and loss of strength in your wrist and hand. [2]

Diabetic Ketoacidosis: High blood glucose with the presence of ketones in the urine and bloodstream, often caused by taking too little insulin or during illness. [1]

Dialysis: A method for removing waste from the blood when the kidneys can no longer do the job. [1]

Hyperosmolar: High blood glucose without the presence of ketones. [3]

Hypertension: Abnormally high blood pressure. [4]

Ketones: Chemical substances that the body makes when it doesn't have enough insulin in the blood. When ketones build up in the body for a long time, serious illness or coma can result. [1]

Retinopathy: A disease of the small blood vessels of the retina of the eye in people with diabetes. In this disease, the vessels swell and leak liquid into the retina, blurring the vision and sometimes leading to blindness. [1]

 • **Indirect costs:** $40 billion (disability, work loss, premature mortality)

These data are based on a study conducted by the Lewin Group, Inc., for the American Diabetes Association and are 2002 estimates of both the direct costs (cost of medical care and services) and indirect costs (costs of short-term and permanent disability and of premature death) attributable to diabetes. This study uses a specific cost-of-disease methodology to estimate the health care costs that are due to diabetes.

Spontaneous Abortion: Loss of a fetus due to natural causes. [3]

Stroke: In medicine, a loss of blood flow to part of the brain, which damages brain tissue. Strokes are caused by blood clots and broken blood vessels in the brain. Symptoms include dizziness, numbness, weakness on one side of the body, and problems with talking, writing, or understanding language. The risk of stroke is increased by high blood pressure, older age, smoking, diabetes, high cholesterol, heart disease, atherosclerosis (a build-up of fatty material and plaque inside the coronary arteries), and a family history of stroke. [5]

Source: [1] "Publications and Products," "Take Charge of Your Diabetes," "Glossary," National Center for Chronic Disease Prevention and Health Promotions, Department of Health and Human Services, January 2005; available online at http://www.cdc.gov/diabetes/pubs/tcyd/appendix.htm. [2] "Carpal Tunnel Syndrome," National Women's Health Information Center (NWHIC), a component of the U.S. Department of Health and Human Services (DHHS), Office on Women's Health, June 2005; available online at http://www.4woman.gov/faq/carpal.htm. [3] Editor. [4] "Genetics Home Reference Glossary," a service of the U.S. National Library of Medicine, July 2005; available at http://www.ghr.nlm.nih.gov. [5] "Dictionary of Cancer Terms," National Cancer Institute, cited July 2005; available at http://www.cancer.gov.

Part Two

Diabetes Treatment And Management

Chapter 13

Your Diabetes Health Care Team

Taking care of your diabetes is like a big class project. It takes all of your team members—you, your parents, doctors, certified diabetes educators, dietitians, and mental health pros—to work together to get the job done. In this case, though, instead of ending up with a presentation for history class or a winning science fair project, you'll have a diabetes treatment plan that helps you stay healthy and lets you do all the things you like to do.

When it comes to treating diabetes, you're the most important member of the team. Your parents still play a very important role—think of them as your co-captains—but your diabetes team will help develop a treatment plan that's made just for you. In addition, the team can help you cope with some of the emotions and feelings that people with diabetes have to deal with.

You'll probably come across one or more of the following diabetes health care team members during your checkups.

About This Chapter: Information in this chapter is from "Your Diabetes Health Care Team." This information was provided by TeensHealth, one of the largest resources online for medically reviewed health information written for parents, kids, and teens. For more articles like this one, visit www.TeensHealth.org, or www.KidsHealth.org. © 2005 The Nemours Center for Children's Health Media, a division of The Nemours Foundation.

Doctors

A pediatric endocrinologist (pronounced: pee-dee-ah-trik en-doh-krih-nah-leh-jist) is a doctor who specializes in the diagnosis and treatment of kids and teens with diseases of the endocrine system, such as diabetes and growth disorders. But pediatricians, family practitioners, and other medical doctors can also treat people with diabetes.

Doctors ask detailed questions about how you feel and perform physical exams, which can include checking your eyes, mouth, hands, feet, and blood pressure. They also may check your diabetes records and your blood sugar level, and they may ask you for a urine sample.

Your doctor can help teach you about diabetes and any other health problem you may have. He or she may get treatment suggestions from all of the diabetes health care team members and will then write down everything you need to do to manage your diabetes. This is called a treatment plan or diabetes management plan. Think of your doctor as your diabetes team coach who develops a game plan for managing diabetes. Doctors also write prescriptions for insulin (pronounced: in-suh-lin) and other medications and may refer you to other specialists if you need them.

Don't be afraid to ask your doctor questions and make sure you're able to understand the answers. If you feel uncomfortable asking questions in front of your parents, you can ask to speak to your doctor alone. Your doctor has probably heard it all, so you shouldn't feel embarrassed or ashamed to ask him or her anything that's on your mind.

Certified Diabetes Educators (CDEs)

Certified diabetes educators (pronounced: ser-tuh-fide dye-uh-be-tees eh-dyoo-kay-ters) are people who have special training in helping people manage their diabetes. Someone with the letters CDE after his or her name has passed a national exam certifying him or her as a diabetes educator.

CDEs will teach you what diabetes is and how it affects the body. They also will:

- help you learn how to give yourself insulin injections if you need them.

- manage high and low blood sugar levels.

- adjust your insulin when you're exercising or not feeling well.

- show you how to test blood sugar levels.

- use a blood glucose meter (pronounced: blud gloo-kose me-tur).

- test your home equipment to make sure it's taking accurate readings.

- review your diabetes management goals with you.

- discuss any problems or challenges you may be having with your diabetes.

Dietitians

Registered dietitians are experts in nutrition and meal planning. They can teach you about how food affects your blood sugar levels and make sure you're getting enough food to grow and develop properly.

When you meet with a dietitian, expect to answer a few questions about your eating habits and activity levels. The dietitian will:

- make adjustments to your meal plan based on the types of exercise you do, your lifestyle habits, and any other special events or holidays that may come up.

- suggest some tasty snack ideas.

- help you learn about making healthy food choices.

- explain carbohydrate (pronounced: kar-bo-hi-drate) counting or other meal planning techniques.

- teach you to read food labels and figure out ways to determine the carbohydrate content of foods when food labels aren't available.

Make sure to tell the dietitian if you feel like you're not getting enough to eat, you think you're eating too much, or you're not happy with your food choices.

Mental Health Professionals

Sometimes people feel uncomfortable talking to anyone who has the words "mental health" or "therapist" associated with what they do. But diabetes can be a lot to deal with and talking to someone who's not your mom, dad, or doctor can help.

Mental health professionals can be social workers, psychologists, psychiatrists, or counselors. They're a great resource for people coping with diabetes. Maybe your parents are always on your back about your diabetes, or maybe you're frustrated because you feel embarrassed to give yourself shots at school or you feel different from your friends. If so, these types of team members can help you get through it.

Mental health professionals can help you address any problems you may be dealing with at home or at school, even if they're not related to your diabetes, so don't be afraid to ask for advice. They can also help you come up with ways to help you manage your diabetes, even when you don't want to deal with it.

☞ Remember!!

The most important thing to remember about your diabetes is that you don't have to manage it on your own. You can always count on your team members to help you, and you can always ask questions—the team has lots of experience figuring out ways to help people deal with diabetes.

Chapter 14

Taking Care Of Your Diabetes Every Day

Do four things every day to lower high blood glucose:

• Follow your meal plan.

• Be physically active.

• Take your diabetes medicine.

• Check your blood glucose.

Experts say most people with diabetes should try to keep their blood glucose level as close as possible to the level of someone who doesn't have diabetes. The closer to normal your blood glucose is, the lower your chances are of developing damage to your eyes, kidneys, and nerves. Check with your doctor about the right range for you.

Your health care team will help you learn how to reach your target blood glucose range. Your main health care providers are your doctor, nurse, diabetes educator, and dietitian.

When you see your health care provider, ask lots of questions. Before you leave, be sure you understand everything you need to know about taking care of your diabetes.

About This Chapter: Excerpted from "Your Guide to Diabetes: Type 1 and Type 2," a publication of the National Diabetes Information Clearinghouse (NDIC), a service of the National Institute of Diabetes and Digestive and Kidney Diseases (NIDDK), National Institutes of Health (NIH), February 2005.

A diabetes educator is a health care worker who teaches people how to manage their diabetes. Your educator may be a nurse, a dietitian, or another kind of health care worker. A dietitian is someone who's specially trained to help people plan their meals.

Follow Your Meal Plan

People with diabetes don't need to eat special foods. The foods on your meal plan are good for everyone in your family. Try to eat foods that are low in fat, salt, and sugar and high in fiber such as beans, fruits, vegetables, and grains. Eating right will help you

- reach and stay at a weight that's good for your body.

- keep your blood glucose in a desirable range.

- prevent heart and blood vessel disease.

People with diabetes should have their own meal plan. Ask your doctor to give you the name of a dietitian who can work with you to develop a meal plan. Your dietitian can help you plan meals to include foods that you and your family like to eat and that are good for you too. Ask your dietitian to include foods that are heart-healthy to reduce your risk of heart disease.

If you use insulin:

- follow your meal plan.

- don't skip meals, especially if you've already taken your insulin, because your blood glucose may go too low.

If you don't use insulin:

- follow your meal plan.

- don't skip meals, especially if you take diabetes medicine, because your blood glucose may go too low. It may be better to eat several small meals during the day instead of one or two big meals.

Be Physically Active

Physical activity is good for your diabetes. Walking, swimming, dancing, riding a bicycle, playing baseball, and bowling are all good ways to be active.

You can even get exercise when you clean house or work in your garden. Physical activity is especially good for people with diabetes because:

- physical activity helps keep weight down.

- physical activity helps insulin work better to lower blood glucose.

- physical activity is good for your heart and lungs.

- physical activity gives you more energy.

Before you begin exercising, talk with your doctor. Your doctor may check your heart and your feet to be sure you have no special problems. If you have high blood pressure or eye problems, some exercises like weightlifting may not be safe. Your health care team can help you find safe exercises.

Try to be active almost every day for a total of about 30 minutes. If you haven't been very active lately, begin slowly. Start with 5 to 10 minutes, and then add more time. Or exercise for 10 minutes, three times a day.

If your blood glucose is less than 100 to 120, have a snack before you exercise.

When you exercise, carry glucose tablets or a carbohydrate snack with you in case you get hypoglycemia (low blood sugar). Wear or carry an identification tag or card saying that you have diabetes.

If you use insulin:

- see your doctor before starting a physical activity program.

- check your blood glucose before, during, and after exercising. Don't exercise when your blood glucose is over 240 or if you have ketones in your urine.

- don't exercise right before you go to sleep, because it could cause hypoglycemia (low blood sugar) during the night.

If you don't use insulin:

- see your doctor before starting a physical activity program.

✎ **What's It Mean?**

Ketone: A chemical produced when there is a shortage of insulin in the blood and the body breaks down body fat for energy. High levels of ketones can lead to diabetic ketoacidosis and coma. Sometimes referred to as ketone bodies.

Ketoacidosis: An emergency condition in which extremely high blood glucose levels, along with a severe lack of insulin, result in the breakdown of body fat for energy and an accumulation of ketones in the blood and urine. Signs of ketoacidosis are nausea and vomiting, stomach pain, fruity breath odor, and rapid breathing. Untreated ketoacidosis can lead to coma and death.

Source: [1] "Diabetes Dictionary," National Diabetes Information Clearinghouse (NDIC), a publication of the National Institute of Diabetes and Digestive and Kidney Diseases (NIDDK), National Institutes of Health (NIH), NIH Publication No. 04-3016, November 2003; available at http://diabetes.niddk.nih.gov/dm/pubs/dictionary.

Take Your Diabetes Medicine Every Day

Insulin and diabetes pills are the two kinds of medicines used to lower blood glucose.

If You Use Insulin

You need insulin if your body has stopped making insulin or if it doesn't make enough. Everyone with type 1 diabetes needs insulin, and many people with type 2 diabetes do too.

Insulin can't be taken as a pill. You'll give yourself shots every day or use an insulin pump. An insulin pump is a small machine that connects to narrow tubing, ending with a needle just under the skin near the abdomen. Insulin is delivered through the needle.

Keep extra insulin in your refrigerator in case you break the bottle you're using. Don't keep insulin in the freezer or in hot places like the glove compartment of your car. Also, keep it away from bright light. Too much heat, cold, or bright light can damage insulin.

If you use a whole bottle of insulin within a month, you can keep that bottle at room temperature. If you don't use a whole bottle of insulin within one month, then store it in the refrigerator.

If You Take Diabetes Pills

If your body makes insulin, but the insulin doesn't lower your blood glucose, you may need diabetes pills. Some pills are taken once a day, and others are taken more often. Ask your health care team when you should take your pills.

Be sure to tell your doctor if your pills make you feel sick or if you have any other problems.

sometimes, people who take diabetes pills may need insulin shots for a while. If you get sick or have surgery, the diabetes pills may no longer work to lower your blood glucose.

You may be able to stop taking diabetes pills if you lose weight. (Always check with your doctor before you stop taking your diabetes pills.) Losing 10 or 15 pounds can sometimes help you reach your target blood glucose level.

If You Don't Use Insulin Or Take Diabetes Pills

Many people with type 2 diabetes don't need insulin or diabetes pills. They can take care of their diabetes by using a meal plan and exercising regularly.

Check Your Blood Glucose As Recommended

You'll want to know how well you're taking care of your diabetes. The best way to find out is to check your blood to see how much glucose is in it. If your blood has too much or too little glucose, you may need a change in your meal plan, exercise plan, or medicine.

☞ **Remember!!**
Diabetes pills don't lower blood glucose all by themselves. You'll still want to follow a meal plan and be active to help lower your blood glucose.

Ask your doctor how often you should check your blood glucose. Some people check their blood glucose once a day. Others do it three or four times a day. You may check before and after eating, before bed, and sometimes in the middle of the night.

Your doctor or diabetes educator will show you how to check your blood using a blood glucose meter.

Take Other Tests For Your Diabetes

Urine Tests

You may need to check your urine if you're sick or if your blood glucose is over 240. A urine test will tell you if you have ketones in your urine. Your body makes ketones when there isn't enough insulin in your blood. Ketones can make you very sick. Call your doctor right away if you find moderate or large amounts of ketones, along with high blood glucose levels, when you do a urine test. You may have a serious condition called ketoacidosis. If it isn't treated, it can cause death. Signs of ketoacidosis are vomiting, weakness, fast breathing, and a sweet smell on the breath. Ketoacidosis is more likely to develop in people with type 1 diabetes.

You can buy strips for testing ketones at a drug store. Your doctor or diabetes educator will show you how to use them.

The A1C Test

Another test for blood glucose, the A1C, also called the hemoglobin A1C test, shows what your overall blood glucose was for the past 3 months. It shows how much glucose is sticking to your red blood cells. The doctor does this test to see what your blood glucose is most of the time. Have this test done at least twice a year.

Ask your doctor what your A1C test showed. A result of under 7 usually means that your diabetes treatment is working well and your blood glucose is under control. If your A1C is 8 or above, it means that your blood glucose may be too high. You'll then have a greater chance of getting diabetes problems, like kidney damage. You may need a change in your meal plan, physical activity plan, or diabetes medicine.

Talk with your doctor about what your target should be. Even if your A1C is higher than your target, remember that every step toward your goal helps reduce your risk of diabetes problems.

Keep Daily Records

Write down the results of your blood glucose checks every day. You may also want to write down what you ate, how you felt, and whether you exercised.

By keeping daily records of your blood glucose checks, you can tell how well you're taking care of your diabetes. Show your blood glucose records to your health care team. They can use your records to see whether you need changes in your diabetes medicines or in your meal plan. If you don't know what your results mean, ask your health care team.

☞ Remember!!

- **Follow your diabetes food plan.** If you do not have one, ask your health care team.

- **Eat the right portions of healthy foods:** fruits and vegetables (5 to 9 servings a day), fish, lean meats, dry beans, whole grains, and low-fat milk and cheese.

- **Eat foods that have less salt and fat.**

- **Get 30 to 60 minutes of activity** on most days of the week.

- **Stay at a healthy weight**—by being active and eating the right amounts of healthy foods.

- **Stop smoking**—seek help to quit.

- **Take medicines** the way your doctor tells you. Ask if you need aspirin to prevent a heart attack or stroke.

- **Check your feet every day** for cuts, blisters, red spots, and swelling. Call your health care team right away about any sores that won't heal.

- **See your dentist** at least twice a year. Tell the dentist you have diabetes.

- **Check your blood glucose** the way your doctor tells you to.

Things to write down every day in your record book are:

- results of your blood glucose checks.

- your diabetes medicines: times and amounts taken.

- if your blood glucose was very low.

- if you ate more or less food than you usually do.

- if you were sick.

- if you found ketones in your urine.

- what kind of physical activity you did and for how long.

If you use insulin, keep a daily record of:

- your blood glucose numbers.

- the times of the day you took your insulin.

- the amount and type of insulin you took.

- whether you had ketones in your urine.

If you don't use insulin, keep a daily record of:

- your blood glucose numbers.

- the times of the day you took your diabetes pills.

- your physical activity.

✔ Quick Tip

Create a plan to deal with diabetes. Use these tips to keep at it.

- Make a list of all your reasons to control your diabetes for life.

- Set goals you can reach and break a big goal into small steps.

- Make changes that you can stick with.

- Try to figure out what tempts you to slip up in reaching your goals. Decide now how you will handle these events next time.

- Reward yourself for staying in control. Spend time with a friend or go to a movie.

- Ask for a little help from friends or family when you're down or need someone to talk to.

- Learn to manage setbacks. Admit that you've slipped and learn what you can from it and move on.

- Don't be too hard on yourself. Work towards a healthy future.

Chapter 15

Glucose Meters And Diabetes Management

When people with diabetes can control their blood sugar (glucose), they are more likely to stay healthy. People with diabetes use two kinds of management devices: glucose meters and other diabetes management tests. Glucose meters help people with diabetes check their blood sugar at home, school, work, and play. Other blood and urine tests reveal trends in diabetes management and help identify diabetes complications.

Self-Monitoring Of Blood Glucose

The process of monitoring one's own blood glucose with a glucose meter is often referred to as self-monitoring of blood glucose or "SMBG." Portable glucose meters are small battery-operated devices.

To test for glucose with a typical glucose meter, place a small sample of blood on a disposable test strip and place the strip in the meter. The test strips are coated with chemicals (glucose oxidase, dehydrogenase, or hexokinase) that combine with glucose in blood. The meter measures how much glucose is present. Meters do this in different ways. Some measure the amount of electricity that can pass through the sample. Others measure how much light reflects from it. The meter displays the glucose level as a number.

About This Chapter: Excerpted from "Glucose Meters & Diabetes Management," U.S. Food and Drug Administration (FDA), Department of Health and Human Services, June 2005.

Several new models can record and store a number of test results. Some models can connect to personal computers to store test results or print them out.

Choosing A Glucose Meter

At least 25 different meters are commercially available.

They differ in several ways including the following:

• Amount of blood needed for each test

• Testing speed

• Overall size

• Ability to store test results in memory

• Cost of the meter

• Cost of the test strips used

Newer meters often have features that make them easier to use than older models. Some meters allow you to get blood from places other than your fingertip (Alternative Site Testing). Some new models have automatic timing, error codes and signals, or barcode readers to help with calibration. Some meters have a large display screen or spoken instructions for people with visual impairments.

Using Your Glucose Meter

Diabetes care should be designed for each individual patient. Some patients may need to test (monitor) more often than others do. How often you use your glucose meter should be based on the recommendation of your health care provider. Self-monitoring of blood glucose (SMBG) is recommended for all people with diabetes, but especially for those who take insulin. The role of SMBG has not been defined for people with stable type 2 diabetes treated only with diet.

> **♣ It's A Fact!!**
> As a general rule, the American Diabetes Association (ADA) recommends that most patients with type 1 diabetes test glucose three or more times per day.

✎ What's It Mean?

Albumin: The main protein in blood plasma. Low levels of serum albumin occur in people with malnutrition, inflammation, and serious liver and kidney disease. [1]

Gestational Diabetes: A type of diabetes mellitus that develops only during pregnancy and usually disappears upon delivery, but increases the risk that the mother will develop diabetes later. GDM is managed with meal planning, activity, and, in some cases, insulin. [2]

Hyperglycemia: Excessive blood glucose. Fasting hyperglycemia is blood glucose above a desirable level after a person has fasted for at least 8 hours. Postprandial hyperglycemia is blood glucose above a desirable level 1 to 2 hours after a person has eaten. [2]

Hypoglycemia: A condition that occurs when one's blood glucose is lower than normal, usually less than 70 mg/dL. Signs include hunger, nervousness, shakiness, perspiration, dizziness or light-headedness, sleepiness, and confusion. If left untreated, hypoglycemia may lead to unconsciousness. Hypoglycemia is treated by consuming a carbohydrate-rich food such as a glucose tablet or juice. It may also be treated with an injection of glucagon if the person is unconscious or unable to swallow. Also called an insulin reaction. [2]

Sickle Cell Anemia: A blood disorder passed down from parents to children. It involves problems in the red blood cells. Normal red blood cells are round and smooth and move through blood vessels easily. Sickle cells are hard and have a curved edge. These cells cannot squeeze through small blood vessels. They block the organs from getting blood. Your body destroys sickle red cells quickly, but it can't make new red blood cells fast enough—a condition called anemia. [3]

Source: [1] "Dictionary of Cancer Terms," National Cancer Institute, cited August 2005; available at http://www.cancer.gov. [2] "Diabetes Dictionary," National Diabetes Information Clearinghouse (NDIC), a publication of the National Institute of Diabetes and Digestive and Kidney Diseases (NIDDK), National Institutes of Health (NIH), NIH Publication No. 04-3016, November 2003; available at http://diabetes.niddk.nih.gov/dm/pubs/dictionary. [3] "NWHIC Web Site Glossary," U.S. Department of Health and Human Services, Office on Women's Health, January 2005; available at www.4woman.gov/Glossary.

Pregnant women taking insulin for gestational diabetes should test two times per day. ADA does not specify how often people with type 2 diabetes should test their glucose, but testing often helps control.

Often, self-monitoring plans direct you to test your blood sugar before meals, 2 hours after meals, at bedtime, at 3 a.m., and anytime you experience signs or symptoms. You should test more often when you change medications, when you have unusual stress or illness, or in other unusual circumstances.

Learning To Use Your Glucose Meter

Not all glucose meters work the same way. Since you need to know how to use your glucose meter and interpret its results, you should get training from a diabetes educator. The educator should watch you test your glucose to make sure you can use your meter correctly. This training is better if it is part of an overall diabetes education program.

The Food and Drug Administration (FDA) requires that glucose meters and the strips used with them have instructions for use. You should read carefully the instructions for both the meter and its test strips. Meter instructions are found in the user manual. Keep this manual to help you solve any problems that may arise. Many meters use error codes when there is a problem with the meter, the test strip, or the blood sample on the strip. You will need the manual to interpret these error codes and fix the problem.

> **✔ Quick Tip**
> **Instructions For Using Glucose Meters**
>
> The following are the general instructions for using a glucose meter:
>
> 1. Wash hands with soap and warm water and dry completely, or clean the area with alcohol and dry completely.
>
> 2. Prick the fingertip with a lancet.
>
> 3. Hold the hand down and hold the finger until a small drop of blood appears; catch the blood with the test strip.
>
> 4. Follow the instructions for inserting the test strip and using the SMBG meter.
>
> 5. Record the test result.

You can get information about your meter and test strips from several different sources. Your user manual should include a toll free number in case you have questions or problems. If you have a problem and can't get a response from this number, contact your healthcare provider or a local emergency room for advice. Also, the manufacturer of your meter should have a website. Check this website regularly to see if it lists any issues with the function of your meter.

New devices are for sale such as laser lancets and meters that can test blood taken from alternative sites of the body other than fingertips. Since new devices are used in new ways and often have new use restrictions, you must review the instructions carefully.

Important Features Of Glucose Meters

There are several features of glucose meters that you need to understand so you can use your meter and understand its results. These features are often different for different meters. You should understand the features of your own meter.

Measurement Range. Most glucose meters are able to read glucose levels over a broad range of values from as low as 0 to as high as 600 mg/dL. Since the range is different among meters, interpret very high or low values carefully. Glucose readings are not linear over their entire range. If you get an extremely high or low reading from your meter, you should first confirm it with another reading. You should also consider checking your meter's calibration.

Whole Blood Glucose Vs. Plasma Glucose. Glucose levels in plasma (one of the components of blood) are generally 10–15% higher than glucose measurements in whole blood (and even more after eating). This is important because home blood glucose meters measure the glucose in whole blood while most lab tests measure the glucose in plasma. There are many meters on the market now that give results as "plasma equivalent". This allows patients to easily compare their glucose measurements in a lab test and at home. Remember that this is just the way that the measurement is presented to you. All portable blood glucose meters measure the amount of glucose in whole blood. The meters that give "plasma equivalent" readings have a built in algorithm that translates the whole blood measurement to make it seem like the result that would be obtained on a plasma sample. It is important for you and your healthcare provider to know whether your meter gives its results as "whole blood equivalent" or "plasma equivalent."

Cleaning. Some meters need regular cleaning to be accurate. Clean your meter with soap and water, using only a dampened soft cloth to avoid damage to sensitive parts. Do not use alcohol (unless recommended in the instructions), cleansers with ammonia, glass cleaners, or abrasive cleaners. Some meters do not require regular cleaning but contain electronic alerts indicating when you should clean them. Only the manufacturer can clean other meters.

Display Of High And Low Glucose Values. Part of learning how to operate a meter is understanding what the meter results mean. Be sure you know how high and low glucose concentrations are displayed on your meter.

Factors That Affect Glucose Meter Performance

The accuracy of your test results depends partly on the quality of your meter and test strips and your training. Other factors can also make a difference in the accuracy of your results.

Hematocrit. Hematocrit is the amount of red blood cells in the blood. Patients with higher hematocrit values will usually test lower for blood glucose than patients with normal hematocrit. Patients with lower hematocrit values will test higher. If you know that you have abnormal hematocrit values you should discuss its possible effect on glucose testing (and HbA1C testing) with your health care provider. Anemia and sickle cell anemia are two conditions that affect hematocrit values.

Other Substances. Many other substances may interfere with your testing process. These include uric acid (a natural substance in the body that can be more concentrated in some people with diabetes), glutathione (an anti-oxidant also called GSH), and ascorbic acid (vitamin C). You should check the package insert for each meter to find what substances might affect its testing accuracy, and discuss your concerns with your health care provider.

Altitude, Temperature And Humidity. Altitude, room temperature, and humidity can cause unpredictable effects on glucose results. Check the meter and test strip package insert for information on these issues. Store and handle the meter and test strips according to the instructions.

Third-Party Test Strips. Third party or "generic glucose reagent strips" are test strips developed as a less expensive option than the strips that the manufacturer intended the meter to be used with. They are typically developed by copying the original strips. Although these strips may work on the meter listed on the package, they could look like strips used for other meters. Be sure the test strip you use is compatible with your glucose meter.

Sometimes manufacturers change their meters and their test strips. These changes are not always communicated to the third-party strip manufacturers. This can make third-party strips incompatible with your meter without your knowledge. Differences can involve the amount, type, or concentration of the chemicals (called "reagents") on the test strip, or the actual size and shape of the strip itself. Meters are sensitive to these features of test strips and may not work well or consistently if they are not correct for a meter. If you are unsure whether or not a certain test strip will work with your meter, contact the manufacturer of your glucose meter.

Making Sure Your Meter Works Properly

You should perform quality control checks to make sure that your home glucose testing is accurate and reliable. Several things can reduce the accuracy of your meter reading even if it appears to still work. For instance, the meter may have been dropped or its electrical components may have worn out. Humidity or heat may damage test strips. It is even possible that your testing technique may have changed slightly. Quality control checks should be done on a regular basis according to the meter manufacturer's instructions. There are two kinds of quality control checks:

Check Using "Test Quality Control Solutions" Or "Electronic Controls". Test quality control solutions and electronic controls are both used to check the operation of your meter. Test quality control solutions check the accuracy of the meter and test strip. They may also give an indication of how well you use your system. Electronic controls only check that the meter is working properly.

Test quality control solutions have known glucose values. Essentially, when you run a quality control test, you substitute the test solution for blood. The difference is that you know what the result should be.

To test your meter with a quality control solution, follow the instructions that accompany the solution. These will guide you to place a certain amount of solution on your test strip and run it through your meter. The meter will give you a reading for the amount of glucose in the sample. Compare this number to the number listed on the test quality control solution. If the results of your test match the values given in the quality control solution labeling, you can be assured the entire system (meter and test strip) is working properly. If results are not correct, the system may not be accurate—contact the manufacturer for advice.

Manufacturers sometimes include quality control solution with their meter. However, most often you must order it separately from a manufacturer or pharmacy.

Some glucose meters also use electronic controls to make sure the meter is working properly. With this method, you place a cartridge or a special "control" test strip in the meter and a signal will appear to indicate if the meter is working.

Take Your Meter With You To The Health Care Provider's Office. This way you can test your glucose while your health care provider watches your technique to make sure you are using the meter correctly. Your healthcare provider will also take a sample of blood and evaluate it using a routine laboratory method. If values obtained on the glucose meter match the laboratory method, you and your healthcare provider will see that your meter is working well and that you are using good technique. If results do not match the laboratory method results, then results you get from your meter may be inaccurate and you should discuss the issue with your healthcare provider and contact the manufacturer if necessary.

New Technologies: Alternative Site Testing

Some glucose meters allow testing blood from alternative sites, such as the upper arm, forearm, base of the thumb, and thigh.

Sampling blood from alternative sites may be desirable, but it may have some limitations. Blood in the fingertips show changes in glucose levels more quickly than blood in other parts of the body. This means that alternative site test results may be different from fingertip test results not because of the meter's ability to test accurately, but because the actual glucose concentration can be different. FDA believes that further research is needed to better understand these differences in test values and their possible impact on the health of people with diabetes.

Glucose concentrations change rapidly after a meal, insulin, or exercise. Glucose levels at the alternative site appear to change more slowly than in the fingertips. Because of this concern, FDA has now requested that manufacturers either show their device is not affected by differences between alternative site and fingertip blood samples during times of rapidly changing glucose, or alert users about possible different values at these times.

Recommended labeling precautions include these statements:

- Alternative site results may be different than the fingertip when glucose levels are changing rapidly (e.g. after a meal, taking insulin, or during or after exercise).

- Do not test at an alternative site, but use samples taken from the fingertip, if:

  - you think your blood sugar is low.

  - you are not aware of symptoms when you become hypoglycemic, or

  - the site results do not agree with the way you feel.

Minimally Invasive And Non-Invasive Glucose Meters

Researchers are exploring new technologies for glucose testing that avoid fingersticks. One of these is based on near-infrared spectroscopy for measurement of glucose. Essentially, this amounts to measuring glucose by shining a beam of light on the skin. It is painless. There are increasing numbers of reports in the scientific literature on the challenges, strengths, and weaknesses of this and other new approaches to testing glucose without fingersticks.

The FDA has approved one "minimally invasive" meter and one "non-invasive" glucose meter. Neither of these should replace standard glucose testing. They are used to obtain additional glucose values between fingerstick tests. Both devices require daily calibration using standard fingerstick glucose measurements and both remain the subject of continuing studies to find how they are best used as tools for diabetes management.

MiniMed Continuous Glucose Monitoring System. The MiniMed system consists of a small plastic catheter (very small tube) inserted just under the skin. The catheter collects small amounts of liquid that is passed through a biosensor to measure the amount of glucose present.

MiniMed is intended for occasional use and to discover trends in glucose levels during the day. It does not give you readings for individual tests, and therefore you can't use it for typical day-to-day monitoring. The device collects measurements over a 72-hour period and then must be downloaded by the patient or healthcare provider. Understanding trends over time might help patients know the best time to do their standard fingerstick tests. You need a prescription to buy MiniMed.

Cygnus GlucoWatch Biographer. GlucoWatch is worn on the arm like a wristwatch. It pulls tiny amounts of fluid from the skin and measures the glucose in the fluid without puncturing the skin. The device requires 3 hours to warm up after it is put on. After this, it can provide up to 3 glucose measurements per hour for 12 hours. Unlike the MiniMed device, the GlucoWatch displays results that can be read by the wearer, although like the MiniMed device, these readings are not meant to be used as replacements for fingerstick-based tests. The results are meant to show trends and patterns in glucose levels rather than report any one result alone. It is useful for detecting and evaluating episodes of hyperglycemia and hypoglycemia. However, you must confirm its results with a standard glucose meter before you take corrective action. You need a prescription to buy GlucoWatch.

Chapter 16

Other Diabetes Management Tests

Glycosylated Hemoglobin

There is hemoglobin in all red blood cells. Hemoglobin is the part of the red blood cell that carries oxygen to the tissues and organs in the body. Hemoglobin combines with blood glucose to make glycosylated hemoglobin or hemoglobin A1c.

Red blood cells store glycosylated hemoglobin slowly over their 120-day life span. When you have high levels of glucose in your blood, your red blood cells store large amounts of glycosylated hemoglobin. When you have normal or near normal levels, your red blood cells store normal or near normal amounts of glycosylated hemoglobin. So, when you measure your glycosylated hemoglobin, you can find out your level of blood glucose, averaged over the last few months.

Doctors have used the glycosylated hemoglobin test for patients with diabetes since 1976. The test is now widely used in the routine monitoring of patients with diabetes mellitus. Your doctor may use this test to see how well you respond to treatment. If you have low test values you probably have lowered risk for having complications from diabetes mellitus.

About This Chapter: Excerpted from "Glucose Meters & Diabetes Management," U.S. Food and Drug Administration (FDA), Department of Health and Human Services, June 2005; available online at http://www.fda.gov/diabetes/glucose.html.

There are now many different ways to measure glycosylated hemoglobin. These tests vary in cost and convenience and you can do some at home. The values (glycosylated hemoglobin index) these tests give can vary too. Talk to your doctor about what your glycosylated hemoglobin index should be.

Patients with diseases affecting hemoglobin, such as anemia, may get wrong values with this test. Vitamins C and E, high levels of lipids, and diseases of the liver and kidneys may all cause the test results to be wrong.

Glycosylated Serum Proteins

Serum proteins, like hemoglobin, combine with glucose to form glycosylated products. Testing these glycosylated products can give information about your glucose control over shorter periods of time than testing glycosylated hemoglobin.

✎ What's It Mean?

Anemia: A condition in which the number of red blood cells is less than normal, resulting in less oxygen being carried to the body's cells.

Ketones: A chemical produced when there is a shortage of insulin in the blood and the body breaks down body fat for energy. High levels of ketones can lead to diabetic ketoacidosis and coma. Sometimes referred to as ketone bodies.

Lipids: A term for fat in the body. Lipids can be broken down by the body and used for energy.

Renal: Having to do with the kidneys. A renal disease is a disease of the kidneys. Renal failure means the kidneys have stopped working.

Serum Proteins: 1. One of the three main nutrients in food. Foods that provide protein include meat, poultry, fish, cheese, milk, dairy products, eggs, and dried beans. 2. Proteins are also used in the body for cell structure, hormones such as insulin, and other functions.

Vascular: Relating to the body's blood vessels.

Source: "Diabetes Dictionary," National Diabetes Information Clearinghouse (NDIC), a publication of the National Institute of Diabetes and Digestive and Kidney Diseases (NIDDK), National Institutes of Health (NIH), NIH Publication No. 04-3016, November 2003; available at http://diabetes.niddk.nih.gov/dm/pubs/dictionary.

☞ Remember!!

It is good to have your glycosylated hemoglobin tested
at least two times a year if you meet your treatment goals or up to
four times a year if you change therapy or do not meet
your treatment goals.

One common test is the fructosamine test. It gives information on your glucose status over a one- to two-week period. High values mean your blood glucose was high over the past two weeks. This test is good for watching short-term changes in your glucose status during pregnancy or after major changes in your therapy. There is no general guideline for when to use this test. Talk to your doctor about whether this test is right for you.

If you have any other disease that can change your serum proteins or if you have large amounts of Vitamin C (ascorbic acid) in your diet, these tests may give wrong values.

Urine Glucose

Only patients who are unable to use blood glucose meters should use urine glucose tests. Testing urine for glucose, which was once the best way for patients to manage their diabetes, has mostly now been replaced by self-monitoring of blood glucose. There are three major drawbacks of urine glucose testing compared to blood testing. First, urine glucose testing will not tell you about low (below 180 mg/dl) glucose levels, since at lower levels glucose does not enter your urine. Second, urine glucose readings change when the volume of your urine changes. Third, your urine glucose level is more of an average value than your blood glucose level. There are several dipstick tests available on the market.

Urine And Blood Ketones

When the body does not have enough insulin, fats are used for fuel instead of glucose. A by-product of burning fats is the production of ketones. Ketones are passed in the urine and can be detected with a urine test.

If you do not have diabetes, you usually have only small amounts of ketones in your blood and urine. If you have diabetes, however, you may have high amounts of ketones and acid, a condition known as ketoacidosis. This condition can cause nausea, vomiting, or abdominal pain and can be life threatening.

You may use urine dipsticks to rapidly and easily measure the ketones in your urine. You dip a dipstick in your urine and follow the instruction on the package to see if you have a high amount of ketones.

If you have type 1 diabetes, are pregnant with preexisting diabetes, or who have diabetes caused by pregnancy (gestational diabetes), you should check your urine for ketones. If you have diabetes and are ill, under stress, or have any symptoms of high ketones, you should also test your urine for ketones.

Results of ketone testing should be interpreted with care. High ketone levels are found when patients are pregnant (in the first morning urine sample), starving, or recovering from a hypoglycemic episode.

There are now tests for measuring ketones in blood that your doctor may use or you can use at home. Some measure a specific ketone (beta-hydroxy-butyric acid) that patients with diabetic ketoacidosis may have.

It is still not known which type of ketone test, blood or urine, offers more aid to people with diabetes.

Microalbumin

One common and extremely serious result of diabetes is kidney failure. Under normal conditions, the kidneys filter toxins from the blood. When the kidney's filtering processes begin to become impaired, protein (microalbumin) begins to spill into the urine. Testing urine for small, yet abnormal amounts of albumin (microalbuminuria) is a common way to detect this condition early, before it can damage your kidneys.

Many urine dipsticks are used to test for large amounts of albumin. To measure a small amount of albumin, which may show an early stage of kidney disease, your health care provider may use specific tests for low levels of albumin (microalbumin tests). To do this test, you may have to collect your urine for several 24-hour periods.

♣ **It's A Fact!!**

The American Diabetes Association (ADA) recommends testing for protein (microalbumin) in the urine in children with type 1 diabetes at puberty or after having diabetes for 5 years.

The ADA recommends that adults with diabetes be tested for microalbumin every 3- to 6-months.

Early detection of micro-albumin is important because it indicates increased risk for both renal and vascular disease. Fortunately, early detection allows for treatments that may delay the beginning of a more serious disease.

Cholesterol

If you have diabetes, you have a higher risk of heart and blood vessel disease (cardiovascular disease). One way to limit this risk is to measure your cholesterol routinely and control it by changing your lifestyle or taking pre-scription drugs. A cholesterol test usually shows your total cholesterol, total triglycerides, and high-density lipoproteins (HDLs).

Chapter 17

Standard Diabetes Control Versus Tight Control

There's a good chance you've heard about tight control, either from your doctor or other member of your diabetes care team, or from things that you've read. In 1993, a study led by the Diabetes Control and Complications Trial (DCCT) showed that when people practiced tight control, keeping their blood sugars as close to normal as possible, they lowered their risk of eye, kidney, and nerve diseases.

What's The Difference Between Tight Control And Standard Control?

For people with type 1 diabetes, standard control usually involves one or two insulin shots a day (usually the same amount of insulin every day) and fewer than 2 daily tests of blood sugar levels. When you practice tight control, you test your blood sugar more frequently each day and decide what your dose of insulin should be depending on your test readings.

"Test my blood sugar even more than I already do? No way. I spend enough time dealing with it already." That's what a lot of people say when they think about changing from standard control to tight control.

♣ It's A Fact!!
Tight Glucose Control Lowers CVD
By About 50 Percent In Diabetes

A significantly lower risk of heart disease can now be added to the list of proven long-term benefits of tight glucose control in people with type 1 diabetes. Researchers announced this finding at the annual scientific meeting of the American Diabetes Association after analyzing cardiovascular (CVD) events such as heart attack, stroke, and angina in patients who took part in the Diabetes Control and Complications Trial (DCCT).

"The longer we follow patients, the more we're impressed by the lasting benefits of tight glucose control," said Saul Genuth, M.D., of Case Western University. Dr. Genuth chairs the follow-up study of DCCT participants called the Epidemiology of Diabetes Interventions and Complications (EDIC) study, which has been looking at the long-term effects of prior intensive versus conventional blood glucose control. "The earlier intensive therapy begins and the longer it is maintained, the better the chances of reducing the debilitating complications of diabetes."

The DCCT was a multicenter study that compared intensive management of blood glucose to conventional control in 1,441 people with type 1 diabetes. Patients 13 to 39 years of age were enrolled in the trial between 1983 and 1989. Those randomly assigned to intensive treatment kept glucose levels as close to normal as possible with at least three insulin injections a day or an insulin pump, guided by frequent self-monitoring of blood glucose. Intensive treatment meant keeping hemoglobin A1c (HbA1c) levels as close as possible to the normal value of 6 percent or less. (The HbA1c blood test reflects a person's average blood sugar over the past 2 to 3 months.) Conventional treatment at the time consisted of one or two insulin injections a day with daily urine or blood glucose testing.

In 1993, researchers announced the DCCT's main findings: intensive glucose control greatly reduces the eye, nerve, and kidney damage of type 1 diabetes. Tight control also lowers the risk of atherosclerosis, according to a study of DCCT participants published in 2003. But what's most remarkable about intensive control, the researchers say, is its long-lasting value.

After 6½ years of the DCCT, HbA1c levels averaged 7 percent in the intensively treated group and 9 percent in the conventionally treated group. When the study ended, the conventionally treated group was encouraged to adopt intensive control and shown how to do it, and researchers began the long-term follow-up of participants. To the researchers' surprise, the benefits of the original 6 years of intensive control have persisted despite the fact that both groups' HbA1c values have leveled off at about 8 percent after a rise in blood glucose in the intensively treated group and a drop in blood glucose in those formerly on conventional treatment.

Among the 1,375 volunteers continuing to participate in the study, the intensively treated patients had less than half the number of CVD events than the conventionally treated group (46 compared to 98 events). Such events included heart attacks, stroke, angina, and coronary artery disease requiring angioplasty or coronary bypass surgery. Thirty-one intensively treated patients (4 percent) and 52 conventionally treated patients (7 percent) had at least one CVD event during the 17 years of follow-up. The average age of participants is 45 years; 53 percent are male.

"The risk of heart disease is about 10 times higher in people with type 1 diabetes than in people without diabetes. It's now clear that high blood glucose levels contribute to the development of heart disease," said David Nathan, M.D., of Massachusetts General Hospital, who co-chaired the DCCT/EDIC research group and presented the results. "The good news is that intensively controlling glucose significantly reduces heart disease as well as damage to the eyes, nerves, and kidneys in people with type 1 diabetes. Tight control is difficult to achieve and maintain, but its advantages are huge."

"The take-home message is that good glucose control should be started as early as possible to delay or prevent serious diabetes-related complications," said Alan D. Cherrington, PhD, president, American Diabetes Association.

Is glucose control just as important for people with type 2 diabetes? "There is a strong and growing body of evidence that everyone with diabetes gains from strict blood glucose control," said Catherine Cowie, PhD, who oversees EDIC for the National Institute of Diabetes and Digestive and Kidney Diseases (NIDDK).

Source: Excerpted from "Tight Glucose Control Lowers CVD by About 50 Percent in Diabetes," NIH News, National Institutes of Health, U.S. Department of Health and Human Services.

There's no doubt about it. Practicing tight control is challenging. It can also be easy to tell yourself that eye, kidney, and nerve disease won't happen to you. Or that even if the complications do affect you, it's a long time away from now, and you're too busy to think about it.

Thinking positively is helpful, but you have to be realistic too. And the truth is that the more successful you are at keeping your blood sugar within the normal range, the better your chances are of avoiding kidney disease, vision problems, and nerve damage, including the loss of arms or legs.

Is Tight Control Beneficial For Everybody With Diabetes?

According to the DCCT study, there are some people who should not practice tight control. These include children under age 13 and people with end-stage kidney disease, severe visual impairment, and coronary artery disease. One of the drawbacks of tight control is that it brings a higher risk of hypoglycemia, or low blood sugar. Accordingly, people who do not experience warning symptoms when their blood sugar becomes too low should not attempt tight control.

People with type 1, who do not fall into the categories listed above, would probably benefit from tight control.

For people with type 2, there is no one answer about whether tight control is beneficial. The best thing to do is to talk with your doctor about your individual case.

Your Health Care Team Is There To Guide You

Talk with your doctor to find out whether you are a good candidate for tight control. If you are, and you decide that you would like to try tight control, you'll have plenty of help. Your diabetes care team will help you learn exactly what you need to do. They'll help you to figure out.

- Exactly what your blood glucose level should be before and after meals.

- How to adjust your insulin to your particular lifestyle—the type of work you do, your level of activity, the kind of food you eat and when you eat it.

- How often you should meet with a dietitian to review what you eat.

- How you should take care of your diabetes if you become pregnant.

- What your family and friends should do if your blood sugar becomes so low that you need their help.

Tight Doesn't Mean Perfect

If you do become committed to practicing tight control, congratulations. You've taken a big step to avoid serious complications in the future. But don't be too hard on yourself if you make a mistake now and then. Keep in mind that any improvement at all will lower your chances of developing complications.

Chapter 18

Medicines For People With Diabetes

Do I need to take diabetes medicine if I have type 1 diabetes?

Type 1 is the type of diabetes that people most often get before 30 years of age. All people with type 1 diabetes need to take insulin because their bodies do not make enough of it. Insulin helps turn food into energy for the body to work.

Do I need to take diabetes medicine if I have type 2 diabetes?

Type 2 is the type of diabetes most people get as adults after the age of 40. But you can also get this kind of diabetes at a younger age.

Healthy eating, exercise, and losing weight may help you lower your blood glucose (also called blood sugar) when you find out you have type 2 diabetes. If these treatments do not work, you may need one or more types of diabetes pills to lower your blood glucose. After a few more years, you may need to take insulin shots because your body is not making enough insulin.

You, your doctor, and your diabetes teacher should always find the best diabetes plan for you.

About This Chapter: Excerpted from "Medicines for People With Diabetes," a publication of the National Diabetes Information Clearinghouse (NDIC), a service of the National Institute of Diabetes and Digestive and Kidney Diseases (NIDDK), National Institutes of Health (NIH), NIH Publication No. 03-4222, December 2002.

Why do I need medicines for type 1 diabetes?

Most people make insulin in their pancreas. If you have type 1 diabetes, your body does not make insulin. Insulin helps glucose from the foods you eat get to all parts of your body and be used for energy.

Because your body no longer makes insulin, you need to take insulin in shots. Take your insulin as your doctor tells you.

Why do I need medicines for type 2 diabetes?

If you have type 2 diabetes, your pancreas usually makes plenty of insulin, but your body cannot correctly use the insulin you make. You might get this type of diabetes if members of your family have or had diabetes. You might also get type 2 diabetes if you weigh too much or do not exercise enough.

After you have had type 2 diabetes for a few years, your body may stop making enough insulin. Then you will need to take diabetes pills or insulin.

What do I need to know about diabetes pills?

Many types of diabetes pills can help people with type 2 diabetes lower their blood glucose. Each type of pill helps lower blood glucose in a different way. The diabetes pill (or pills) you take is from one of these groups. You might know your pill (or pills) by a different name.

- **Sulfonylureas** (SUL-fah-nil-YOO-ree-ahs) stimulate your pancreas to make more insulin.

☞ **Remember!!**
- Diabetes medicines that lower blood glucose never take the place of healthy eating and exercise.
- If your blood glucose gets too low more than a few times in a few days, call your doctor.
- Take your diabetes pills or insulin even if you are sick. If you cannot eat much, call your doctor.

- **Biguanides** (by-GWAN-ides) decrease the amount of glucose made by your liver.

- **Alpha-glucosidase inhibitors** (AL-fa gloo-KOS-ih-dayss in-HIB-it-ers) slow the absorption of the starches you eat.

- **Thiazolidinediones** (THIGH-ah-ZO-li-deen-DYE-owns) make you more sensitive to insulin.

- **Meglitinides** (meh-GLIT-in-ides) stimulate your pancreas to make more insulin.

- **D-phenylalanine** (dee-fen-nel-AL-ah-neen) derivatives help your pancreas make more insulin quickly.

- **Combination oral medicines** put together different kinds of pills.

Your doctor might prescribe one pill. If the pill does not lower your blood glucose, your doctor may:

- ask you to take more of the same pills, or

- add a new pill or insulin, or

- ask you to change to another pill or insulin.

♣ **It's A Fact!!**
What are side effects?

- Side effects are changes that may happen in your body when you take a medicine. When your doctor gives you a new medicine, ask what the side effects might be.

- Some side effects happen just when you start to take the medicine. Then they go away.

- Some side effects happen only once in a while. You may get used to them or learn how to manage them.

- Some side effects will cause you to stop taking the medicine. Your doctor may try another one that doesn't cause you side effects.

What do I need to know about insulin?

If your pancreas no longer makes enough insulin, then you need to take insulin as a shot. You inject the insulin just under the skin with a small, short needle.

Can insulin be taken as a pill?

Insulin is a protein. If you took insulin as a pill, your body would break it down and digest it before it got into your blood to lower your blood glucose.

How does insulin work?

Insulin lowers blood glucose by moving glucose from the blood into the cells of your body. Once inside the cells, glucose provides energy. Insulin lowers your blood glucose whether you eat or not. You should eat on time if you take insulin.

How often should I take insulin?

Most people with diabetes need at least two insulin shots a day for good blood glucose control. Some people take three or four shots a day to have a more flexible diabetes plan.

When should I take insulin?

You should take insulin 30 minutes before a meal if you take regular insulin alone or with a longer-acting insulin. If you take rapid-acting insulin, you should take your shot just before you eat.

Are there several types of insulin?

Yes. There are six main types of insulin. They each work at different speeds. Many people take two types of insulin.

Does insulin work the same all the time?

After a short time, you will get to know when your insulin starts to work, when it works its hardest to lower blood glucose, and when it finishes working.

You will learn to match your mealtimes and exercise times to the time when each insulin dose you take works in your body.

How quickly or slowly insulin works in your body depends on:

- your own response.

- the place on your body where you inject insulin.

- the type and amount of exercise you do and the length of time between your shot and exercise.

Where on my body should I inject insulin?

You can inject insulin into several places on your body. Insulin injected near the stomach works fastest. Insulin injected into the thigh works slowest. Insulin injected into the arm works at medium speed. Ask your doctor or diabetes teacher to show you the right way to take insulin and in which parts of the body to inject it.

How should I store insulin?

- If you use a whole bottle of insulin within 30 days, keep that bottle of insulin at room temperature. On the label, write the date that is 30 days away. That is when you should throw out the bottle with any insulin left in it.

- If you do not use a whole bottle of insulin within 30 days, then store it in the refrigerator all the time.

- If insulin gets too hot or cold, it breaks down and does not work. So, do not keep insulin in very cold places such as the freezer, or in hot places, such as by a window or in the car's glove compartment during warm weather.

- Keep at least one extra bottle of each type of insulin you use in your house. Store extra insulin in the refrigerator.

What are possible side effects of insulin?

- hypoglycemia
- weight gain

Might I take more than one diabetes medicine at a time?

Yes. Your doctor may ask you to take more than one diabetes medicine at a time. Some diabetes medicines that lower blood glucose work well together. Here are examples:

Two Diabetes Pills: If one type of pill alone does not control your blood glucose, then your doctor might ask you to take two kinds of pills. You may take two separate pills or one pill that combines two medicines. Each type of pill has its own way of acting to lower blood glucose. Here are pills used together:

- a sulfonylurea and metformin
- a sulfonylurea and acarbose
- metformin and acarbose
- repaglinide and metformin
- nateglinide and metformin
- pioglitazone and a sulfonylurea
- pioglitazone and metformin
- rosiglitazone and metformin
- rosiglitazone and a sulfonylurea

Diabetes Pills And Insulin: Your doctor might ask you to take insulin and one of these diabetes pills:

- a sulfonylurea
- metformin
- pioglitazone

What should I know about hypoglycemia (low blood sugar)?

Sulfonylureas, meglitinides, D-phenylalanine derivatives, combination oral medicines, and insulin are the types of diabetes medicines that can make blood glucose go too low. Hypoglycemia can happen for many reasons:

- delaying or skipping a meal
- eating too little food at a meal
- getting more exercise than usual
- taking too much diabetes medicine
- drinking alcohol

You know your blood glucose may be low when you feel one or more of the following:

- dizzy or light-headed

- hungry

- nervous and shaky

- sleepy or confused

- sweaty

If you think your blood glucose is low, test it to see for sure. If your blood glucose is at or below 70 mg/dL, have one of these items to get 15 grams of carbohydrate:

- ½ cup (4 oz.) of any fruit juice

- 1 cup (8 oz.) of milk

- 1 or 2 teaspoons of sugar or honey

- ½ cup (4 oz.) of regular soda

- 5 or 6 pieces of hard candy

- glucose gel or tablets (take the amount noted on the package to add up to 15 grams of carbohydrate)

Test your blood glucose again 15 minutes later. If it is still below 70 mg/dL, then eat another 15 grams of carbohydrate. Then test your blood glucose again in 15 minutes.

If you cannot test your blood glucose right away, but you feel symptoms of hypoglycemia, eat one of the items listed above.

If your blood glucose is not low, but you will not eat your next meal for at least an hour, then have a snack with starch and protein. Here are some examples:

- crackers and peanut butter or cheese

- half of a ham or turkey sandwich

- a cup of milk and crackers or cereal

How do I know if my diabetes medicines are working?

Learn to test your blood glucose. Ask your doctor or diabetes teacher about the best testing tools for you and how often to test. After you test your blood glucose, write down your blood glucose test results. Then ask your doctor or diabetes teacher if your diabetes medicines are working. A good blood glucose reading before meals is between 70 and 140 mg/dL.

Ask your doctor or diabetes teacher about how low or how high your blood glucose should get before you take action. For many people, blood glucose is too low below 70 mg/dL and too high above 240 mg/dL.

One other number to know is the result of a blood test your doctor does called the A1C. It shows your blood glucose control during the past 2 to 3 months. For most people, the target for A1C is less than 7 percent.

Chapter 19

The Basic Facts About Insulin

There are many different insulins for many different situations and lifestyles. This chapter should help you and your doctor decide which insulin or insulins are best for you.

Characteristics

The three characteristics of insulin are:

Onset. The length of time before insulin reaches the bloodstream and begins lowering blood glucose.

Peak time. The time during which insulin is at its maximum strength in terms of lowering blood glucose levels.

Duration. How long the insulin continues to lower blood glucose.

Kinds

Here is a brief look at the kinds of insulins available. Remember that each person has his or her unique response to insulin, so the times mentioned here are approximate.

About This Chapter: Information in this chapter is from "Resource Guide 2005." Copyright © 2005 American Diabetes Association. From *Diabetes Forecast*, January 2005. Reprinted with permission from The American Diabetes Association.

Rapid-acting insulins, such as insulin lispro (by Lilly) or insulin aspart (by Novo Nordisk), begin to work about 15 minutes after they are injected, peak in about an hour, and continue to work for 2 to 4 hours. (The Food and Drug Administration [FDA] has approved another rapid-acting insulin called insulin glulisine [Apidra], which is manufactured by Aventis, but it is not yet available to consumers.) People should inject rapid-acting insulins immediately before a meal. (In fact, meals should not be delayed when using insulin lispro or insulin aspart.) Also, because these insulins leave the bloodstream quickly, there is less chance of hypoglycemia (low blood glucose) several hours after the meal. Both insulin lispro and insulin aspart are only available by prescription. Insulin lispro and insulin aspart are very similar in their activity, but you should not use them interchangeably unless advised to do so by your doctor.

After-meal use of rapid-acting insulins may also be of some benefit to children, because their caloric intake is often difficult to predict before meals. After-meal use can also benefit those who have delayed gastroparesis (stomach emptying).

Regular or short-acting insulin (human) usually reaches the bloodstream within 30 minutes after injection. It peaks anywhere from 2 to 3 hours after injection, and is effective for approximately 3 to 6 hours. Typically, the higher the dose of regular insulin, the greater the effect.

Intermediate-acting insulin (human) generally reaches the bloodstream about 2 to 4 hours after it is injected. It peaks 4 to 12 hours later, and is effective for about 12 to 18 hours. The varieties of intermediate-acting insulin include both NPH and lente. These are often used in combination with short-acting insulin.

Long-acting insulin (ultralente) reaches the bloodstream 6 to 10 hours after injection and is usually effective for 18 to 24 hours. It does have peak action, so ultralente does not mimic basal insulin action.

Human ultralente, which is considered to be a long-acting insulin, may be absorbed at different rates in different people. Therefore, for some people, human ultralente functions as an intermediate-acting insulin, while for others, it is long acting.

A long-acting insulin known as insulin glargine (trade name Lantus) was approved for use in April 2000. Insulin glargine has continuous, "peakless" action that mimics natural basal (background) insulin secretion. Although it provides a long-lasting effect, insulin glargine's onset is between 2 to 4 hours— quicker than other long-acting insulins. Insulin glargine has been clinically proven to reduce low blood glucose, especially during the night. Giving it at supper is an important advance for the treatment of children in preventing nocturnal lows.

Insulin glargine is the only long-acting insulin that is clear in appearance. However, insulin glargine must not be mixed with any other type of insulin and should not be administered intravenously.

Many people use both rapid- or short-acting insulins and insulin glargine in an effort to mimic the body's natural insulin secretion. Because insulin glargine has no peak, injections of rapid-acting insulin must be given before all meals to provide bolus coverage for food intake. Both types of insulin are clear in appearance. If you are on this type of insulin therapy, it is very important that you choose the correct dose from the correct vial of insulin. (One distinguishing factor is that insulin glargine vials are taller and narrower than those of other insulins.) Insulin glargine can be injected any time during the day, as long as it is at the same time each day. However, the duration of action may be shorter in young children who may require twice-daily injections.

Premixed insulins are convenient for those who draw up a mixture of NPH and regular in one syringe. Often, the insulin is premixed in a prefilled insulin pen, a portable and accurate means of administering insulin, replacing the traditional vial and syringe.

The most typical mixture is 70 percent NPH and 30 percent regular. A new mixture of 75 percent insulin lispro protamine and 25 percent insulin lispro, known on the market as the Humalog Mix 75/25, combines rapid-acting mealtime insulin and intermediate-acting insulin. Likewise, a new mixture of 70 percent insulin aspart protamine and 30 percent insulin aspart is available.

NovoLog (insulin aspart), Humalog (insulin lispro), NovoLog Mix 70/ 30, and Humalog Mix 75/25 can be given just after the meal if patients are experiencing low blood glucose at mealtimes or are erratic eaters.

Premixed insulin can be helpful for people who have trouble drawing up insulin out of two different bottles and reading the correct directions and dosages. It's also useful for those who have poor eyesight or dexterity and is convenient for people whose diabetes has been stabilized on this combination. Insulin pens are also useful for those with dexterity problems or poor eyesight.

Sources

Today, recombinant DNA human insulins are the most widely used insulins in this country. Through genetic engineering, bacteria or yeast are transformed into little "factories" that produce synthetic human insulin. Years ago, the most commonly used insulins were pork, beef, and beef-pork combinations.

The source of an insulin is important because it affects how quickly an insulin will be absorbed, peak, and last.

Another important point is that insulins from animal sources are more likely to cause allergic reactions. However, many people have taken these insulins for years without problems.

✎ What's It Mean?

Basal Insulin Action: A steady trickle of low levels of longer-acting insulin. [1]

Bolus: An extra amount of insulin taken to cover an expected rise in blood glucose, often related to a meal or snack. [1]

Recombinant DNA: Recombinant DNA molecules are either: 1) molecules which are constructed outside living cells by joining natural or synthetic DNA segments to DNA molecules that can replicate in a living cell; or 2) DNA molecules that result from the replication of those described in 1). [2]

Source: "Diabetes Dictionary," National Diabetes Information Clearinghouse (NDIC), a publication of the National Institute of Diabetes and Digestive and Kidney Diseases (NIDDK), National Institutes of Health (NIH), NIH Publication No. 04-3016, November 2003; available at http://diabetes .niddk.nih.gov/dm/pubs/dictionary. [2] "NIAID Glossary of Funding and Policy Terms and Acronyms," National Institute of Allergy and Infectious Diseases, National Institutes of Health (NIH), June 2005; available at http:// www.niaid.nih.gov/ncn/glossary.

Strength

All insulins come dissolved or suspended in liquids, but the solutions have different strengths. The most commonly used strength in the United States today is U-100. That means it has 100 units of insulin per milliliter of fluid (100 units per cc). Not used in the United States, but still used in Europe and Latin America, is U-40, which has 40 units of insulin per milliliter of liquid.

If you are traveling, it's essential that you purchase the correct strength of insulin. And because different syringes are used for different insulin strengths (for example, U-40 syringes deliver U-40 insulin and U-100 syringes deliver U-100 insulin), it's essential that your syringe match your insulin.

U-500 insulin can be purchased in the United States, but it is rarely used. It is available by prescription only, and must be ordered by the pharmacy from the manufacturer. It usually takes two to three days to obtain this type of insulin, so if you use it, plan ahead.

If you take U-500 insulin, you will have to use a U-100 syringe or a tuberculin syringe, which is designed for very small doses. When discussing your insulin dosage with a new health care provider—for example, if you are in the hospital—be sure to specify that you use U-500 insulin.

Mixing Insulins

Often people will be instructed to take a given amount of rapid-acting and a given amount of another type of insulin. NPH insulins mix easily with regular, insulin aspart, and insulin lispro, and if need be, the syringes may be filled a week in advance. It may be easier to use a premixed insulin if your dose approximates that of the premixed insulins.

Some doctors advise against mixing regular insulin with lente or ultralente insulins because such mixtures may lead to unpredictable results. However, some people have achieved good control with these mixtures. If your doctor suggests that you mix regular and lente or ultralente, be sure to take the injection immediately after mixing. Problems are more likely to occur if the mixture is allowed to sit. The interval between mixing and administration should be standardized for more predictable results.

✔ **Quick Tip**
Consumer Advice

Convenience. In selecting a pharmacy for purchasing your insulin and diabetes supplies, consider one that is close to you and open during the hours you want to shop.

Service. Those who order insulin by mail should consider the effect of shipping during hot summer months in the South or freezing winter months in the North. Ask the distributor how the bottles will be kept cool and inspect the bottles carefully when they arrive.

If you choose to use a local pharmacy, look for one that makes deliveries. This can be helpful when you are ill or busy.

Professional pharmacist. Use a store where a pharmacist is available, and get to know him or her. Make sure the pharmacist will take an interest in your medical needs, be available to answer questions, and tell you what problems to watch for.

Check labels. Don't just ask for "NPH insulin"; look at the full brand name, strength, and kind. In fact, you might bring a used bottle with you to make sure you get the same exact insulin you got before. Then, before you pay, check the insulin label to make sure you have the correct insulin and the correct directions.

Expiration date. Make sure you will be using all the insulin you are buying before its expiration date.

Quantity purchases. Inquire whether buying more than one bottle of insulin at a time would be cheaper than buying it by the bottle. Of course, keep the expiration date in mind.

Keep alert. On the rare occasion that insulin lots must be recalled, check to see if the control number on any of your bottles matches that of the recalled lot.

Price. It does pay to shop around for your insulin. Prices can vary by several dollars a bottle depending on where it's sold. (Note: Don't switch brands or types of insulin without your doctor's advice.) However, it is important to get all of your prescriptions at one pharmacy.

Additives

All insulins have added ingredients. These prevent bacteria from growing and help maintain a neutral balance between acids and bases.

In addition, intermediate- and long-acting insulins also contain ingredients that prolong their actions.

In some rare cases, the additives can bring on an allergic reaction.

Storage And Safety

👉 **Remember!!**

Do not store your insulin at extreme temperatures. Never store insulin in the freezer, in direct sunlight, or in the glove compartment of a car.

Although manufacturers recommend storing your insulin in the refrigerator, injecting cold insulin can sometimes make the injection more painful. To counter that, many providers recommend storing the bottle of insulin you are using at room temperature. Most believe that insulin kept at room temperature will last about a month.

Remember, though, if you buy more than one bottle at a time—a possible money-saver—store the extra bottles in the refrigerator. Then, take out the bottle ahead of time so it is ready for your next injection.

Before you use any insulin, especially if you have had it awhile, check the expiration date. Don't use any insulin beyond its expiration date. And examine the bottle closely to make sure the insulin looks normal before you draw the insulin into the syringe. If you use regular, insulin aspart, insulin lispro, or insulin glargine, make sure the insulin is clear. Check for particles or discoloration of the insulin. If you use NPH, ultralente, or lente, check for "frosting" or crystals in the insulin or on the inside of the bottle, or for small particles or clumps in the insulin. If you find any of these in your insulin, do not use it, and return the unopened bottle to the pharmacy for exchange or refund.

Chapter 20

Insulin Delivery Methods

Syringes...pumps...jet injectors...pens...infusers...they all do the same basic thing—deliver insulin. These items carry insulin through the outermost layer of skin and into fatty tissue so the body can use it. This chapter will also cover injection aids—products designed to make injecting easier. [Note: The first inhaled insulin product was approved by the U.S. Food and Drug Administration in January 2006. See pages 160 and 162 for more information.]

Syringes

Today's syringes are smaller and have finer points and special coatings that work to make injecting as easy and painless as possible. When insulin injections are done properly, most people discover they are relatively painless.

Check with your doctor or diabetes educator and test several brands before you buy. Your equipment should suit your needs.

Questions to ask:

• Does the syringe dose match your insulin strength? If you take U-100 insulin, use U-100 syringes. (Note: All insulin syringes in the United States take U-100 insulin.)

About This Chapter: Information in this chapter is from "Resource Guide 2005." Copyright © 2005 American Diabetes Association. From *Diabetes Forecast*, January 2005. Reprinted with permission from The American Diabetes Association.

- Does your syringe match your insulin dosage? If you take 30 units or less of insulin, you may use the 3/10-cc syringe. The ½-cc syringe may be used by those taking 50 units or less, and the 1-cc syringe is designed for those needing up to 100 units of insulin. If your insulin needs have been increasing, you might want to buy syringes that give you an opportunity to increase your dose if need be. For example, if you take 29 units, consider buying a 50-unit syringe. Using a syringe that more closely matches your dose may help you more accurately draw up your insulin. If you are changing the syringe you use, check dosage lines carefully. In some syringes, one line is equal to one unit of insulin, but in others, each line is equal to two units of insulin.

- Be familiar with the gauge of your needle and what it means. The higher the gauge number of your needle, the thinner it is.

- Can you easily draw up your dosage in a particular syringe? Does the syringe barrel have the kind of markings you can read easily, or are they too close together? Does having a plunger that's a different color make it easier for you?

- Would a shorter needle be a better choice for you? Some syringes now have shorter needles that many people find to be more comfortable. However, the depth of the injection can change the rate of absorption. Ask your doctor or diabetes educator to assess whether this would be a good alternative to your current syringe.

- Does this brand come packaged as you prefer?

Cost is another factor because many stores use insulin syringes as key sale items. Shop around for a good price, but ask yourself: Is giving up a good local pharmacist to save $2 at an out-of-the-way store worth the money?

You may be interested in reusing your syringes. Most manufacturers do not recommend this, and there may be some increased risk to patients (i.e., needle dullness causing discomfort, possible infection, or tissue damage). While this practice remains controversial, many patients reuse syringes without any problems. Once again, your health care team can advise you on the practice. (Pen needles, however, should always be removed immediately after use; when left in place, they create an open passage to the insulin chamber. The open passage may allow bacteria into the chamber or fluid to leak out, which may alter the strength of the insulin.)

Pumps

The insulin pump is not an artificial pancreas (because you still have to monitor your blood glucose level), but pumps can help some people achieve better control, and many people prefer this continuous system of insulin delivery to injections.

Insulin pumps are computerized devices, about the size of a call-beeper that you can wear on your belt or in your pocket. They deliver insulin in two ways: in a steady, measured and continuous dose (the "basal" insulin) and as a surge ("bolus") dose, at your direction, around mealtime. Doses are delivered through a flexible plastic tube called a catheter. With the aid of a small needle, the catheter is inserted through the skin into the fatty tissue and is taped in place. In the newer products, the needle is removed and only a soft catheter remains in place.

Remember!!
Always follow appropriate guidelines when disposing of your syringes and lancets. Some states have very specific laws governing disposal of such items, while others lack guidelines. Even if no guidelines exist, you should be considerate of those who could possibly come in contact with used syringes and lancets. Used syringes and lancets can be safely placed in a puncture-proof container that can be sealed shut before it is placed in the trash. (Label the container "USED SHARPS" with a heavy magic marker.)

If you use Humalog or NovoLog, which are rapid-acting insulins, you can direct your pump to release a bolus dose close to mealtime to blunt the rise in blood glucose after a meal. If you use regular insulin, you would usually take the bolus dose about 30 minutes before you eat.

Because the pump also releases incredibly small doses of insulin continuously, this delivery system most closely mimics the body's normal release of insulin. Also, pumps deliver very precise insulin doses for different times of day, which in many instances are necessary to correct for situations like the dawn phenomenon, the rise of blood glucose that occurs in the hours before and after waking.

Many people have chosen the insulin pump because it enables them to enjoy a more flexible lifestyle. To use a pump, however, you must be willing to check your blood glucose frequently and learn how to make adjustments in insulin, food, and physical activity in response to those test results. (These things should be done with insulin injections as well.)

You'll want to check with your insurance carrier before you buy a pump and all the supplies. Although most carriers do cover these items, some do not. (Please note: Medicare now covers pumps and supplies for people with diabetes [both type 1 and type 2] who meet its eligibility requirements, including those regarding fasting C-peptide levels.)

If you are interested in using a pump, talk to your health care team.

Injection Aids And Alternatives

This category includes devices that make giving injections easier as well as syringe alternatives.

Make sure that the injection aid you purchase works with your brand of syringe and needle length. Some injection aids have adapters for short needles.

Insertion aids. These devices accelerate needle insertion into the skin. Some even aid in pushing down the plunger. Most are spring-loaded and hide the needle from view.

✔ **Quick Tip**
Talk with your doctor or diabetes educator about injection aids and alternatives. Oftentimes, they will make sample products available to you before you make a purchase. You'll want to look for an item that is easy for you to use and is durable. Some items require more skill and dexterity on the part of the user than others do, so try several before you buy.

Syringe alternatives. At present, this category includes insulin pens, infusers, and jet injectors.

Carrying around an insulin pen is like having an old-fashioned cartridge pen in your pocket—only instead of a writing point, there's a needle, and instead of an ink cartridge, there's an insulin cartridge. (See note above on removing pen needles after use.) There are even disposable insulin pens now available. The devices are convenient, accurate, and often used by people on a multidose regimen. Insulin cartridges may come in limited total capacities of regular, NPH, insulin lispro, or 70/30 or 75/25 premixed insulin. They are particularly useful for people whose coordination or vision is impaired, or for people who are on the go.

If you are using a pen with NPH, 70/30, or 75/25, it is important to tip the pens back and forth at least 10 times to ensure the insulin is well mixed.

Infusers create "portals" into which you inject insulin. With an infuser, a needle or catheter is inserted into subcutaneous tissues and remains taped in place, usually on the abdomen, for 48–72 hours. The insulin is injected into it, rather than directly through the skin into the fatty tissue. Some people are prone to infections with this type of product, so be sure to discuss the necessary cleaning procedures with your health care team.

Jet injectors release a tiny jet stream of insulin, which is forced through the skin with pressure, not a puncture. These devices have no needles. However, they can sometimes cause bruising. You will need to work with your health care team to ensure good blood glucose control while you adjust to one of these devices.

You'll want to ask manufacturers about training on the use of a jet injector, as well as how to clean it and how to troubleshoot. If jet injectors interest you, discuss their use with your health care team. Before buying, check to be sure that your insurance covers jet injectors.

Aids For People With Visual Impairments

There are several products designed to make injections easier for people who are visually impaired. Some products handle more than one task.

Non-visual insulin measurement. Helps you measure an accurate dose of insulin. Some "click" at each 1- or 2-unit increment of insulin.

Needle guides and vial stabilizers. Help you insert the needle into the correct insulin vial for drawing up an injection.

Syringe magnifiers. Enlarge the measure marks on a syringe barrel.

It's important to note that some of these aids fit only with specific brands of syringes, so check to be sure the product you want works with your syringe.

Chapter 21

Tips For Site Rotation For Insulin Injections

When it comes to insulin, where you inject is just as important as how much and when. For years, people who inject insulin have been advised to rotate or change their injection sites regularly. That advice still stands, even though times have changed and some of the original reasons for doing so no longer hold.

Insulin has come a long way in 25 years. Up until human insulins were introduced in the early 1980s, insulin was derived from cows and pigs. It was important to switch injection sites at random to avoid a condition called lipoatrophy. Lipoatrophy is a thinning or pitting of the fat layer under the skin where repeated injections are given, and it's caused by an immune response to animal insulins, particularly insulins derived from cows. With today's more purified human insulins and analogs, lipoatrophy is not the problem that it once was, and random site selection is no longer recommended.

However, if you take insulin by injection, you should still move your injection sites around. But not randomly; instead, today's educators recommend an orderly and consistent method of site rotation. That's because repeated injections in the same site can cause fat to accumulate over a period of time.

About This Chapter: "Tips For Site Rotation," by Terry Lumber, RN, CNS, CDE, BC-ADM. Copyright © 2004 American Diabetes Association. From *Diabetes Forecast*, July 2004. Reprinted with permission from The American Diabetes Association.

Think of it as a callus. Your skin can become lumpy, bumpy, or thickened when you inject at the same site too often. This can cause your blood glucose levels to fluctuate because the accumulation of fat reduces and delays the absorption of insulin.

Each Site Is Different

Insulin should always be injected into subcutaneous fat, the fatty tissue that lies right under the skin and right above the layer of muscle. Although there is subcu-

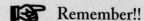 **Remember!!**

Using site rotation, you can avoid overusing your injection sites and keep your blood glucose in better control.

taneous fat all over your body, it's important not to inject insulin too close to large blood vessels and nerves, so only certain sites will do. Insulin is absorbed the most quickly in the abdomen, followed by the outer part of your upper arms, then the outer parts of your thighs. It's absorbed the most slowly in the hips and buttocks. The long-acting insulin glargine (Lantus) is the exception to the rule. No significant difference in absorption between sites has been observed with insulin glargine. However, if you use insulin glargine, you should still rotate sites to avoid the accumulation of fat underneath your skin.

If you inject insulin into your abdomen, make sure the injection site is at least two inches away from your belly button. Do not inject insulin into your inner thigh because of the concentration of blood vessels and nerves in that area.

Things To Remember

Developing a site rotation plan is a team effort. Work with your diabetes educator or diabetes care provider to find the best site rotation plan for you. Your plan should be based on your insulin regimen, your body type, and your personal preferences.

Here are some things to keep in mind when discussing site rotation with your care provider.

The abdomen works. It's okay to use only your abdomen as long as you rotate your injection sites within the area. This method allows for the most consistent absorption.

Timing is everything. If you inject into more than one area, try to give your injections in the same area at the same time each day. For example, you can take your morning insulin in your abdomen and your afternoon or evening insulin in your thighs. This will also give you some consistency in absorption.

Different sites can be used for different insulins. Each site can be designated for a specific insulin. For example, you might take rapid-acting (pre-meal) insulin in your abdomen and long-acting insulin in your thighs or buttocks.

Distance matters. When rotating sites within one injection area, keep injections about an inch (or two finger widths) apart.

Exercise affects absorption. Massage or exercise that occurs around the time of the injection may speed up absorption because of increased circulation to the injection site. If you plan on strenuous physical activity shortly after injecting, don't inject your insulin in an area affected by the exercise. For example, if you plan to play tennis, don't inject into your racquet arm. If you plan to walk, jog, or run, don't inject into your thighs.

Temperature counts. The temperature outdoors or in a room can affect insulin absorption because it affects your circulation. Hot temperatures speed absorption because they increase circulation at the injection site. Cold temperatures have the opposite effect.

Damaged areas are off-limits. Do not inject into scar tissue or areas with broken blood vessels or varicose veins. Scar tissue may interfere with absorption. Avoid areas with varicose veins and broken blood vessels to avoid mistakenly injecting directly into a blood vessel. Insulin should always be injected into fatty tissue.

Consistency is key. Whatever site rotation you use, be consistent. Do not randomly inject your insulin from site to site (for example, from arm to thigh to abdomen).

A site rotation plan will help you avoid inconsistent insulin absorption and fluctuating blood glucose levels. Once you have devised a plan with your health care provider, keep track of how well it works. If it's not working as well as you would like, don't be afraid to call your health care team. Don't quit until you've found the system that works right for you.

Chapter 22

How To Throw Out Used Insulin Syringes And Lancets

People living in the United States use more than one billion (1,000,000,000) syringes, needles, and lancets each year to take care of their diabetes. This chapter shows you the safe way to handle and throw out used insulin syringes and lancets at home.

It's simple. The easy directions on the following pages show you how to protect your family and waste handlers from injury—and help keep the environment clean and safe.

Remember!!

Keep your container out of reach of small children and pets.

While you are reading this, keep in mind that your state, county, or town may have special rules about how to dispose of syringes and lancets. They may also have a special collection center for these items. You should ask your doctor, diabetes educator, or community representative how to find out about any rules or collection programs in your area.

People with insulin-dependent diabetes know how important syringes and lancets are for controlling their diabetes and staying healthy. Most people

About This Chapter: Information in this chapter is excerpted from "Handle With Care: How To Throw Out Used Insulin Syringes and Lancets At Home," a publication of the United States Environmental Protection Agency, September 1999, updated November 2003.

♣ It's A Fact!!
New Information About Disposing of Medical Sharps

The Coalition for Safe Community Needle Disposal, comprised of medical, government, and waste association and private sector companies, is working with the Environmental Protection Agency to evaluate and promote alternative disposal methods for used needles and other medical sharps.

Improper management of discarded needles and other sharps can pose a health risk to the public and waste workers. For example, discarded needles may expose waste workers to potential needle stick injuries and potential infection when containers break open inside garbage trucks or needles are mistakenly sent to recycling facilities. Janitors and housekeepers also risk injury if loose sharps poke through plastic garbage bags. Used needles can transmit serious diseases, such as HIV and hepatitis.

The Coalition has identified several types of safe disposal programs for self-injectors. Instead of placing sharps in the trash, self-injectors are encouraged to use any of these alternative disposal methods:

Drop Box Or Supervised Collection Sites

Sharps users can take their own sharps containers filled with used needles to appropriate collection sites: doctors' offices, hospitals, pharmacies, health departments, or fire stations. Services are free or have a nominal fee. Check with your pharmacist or other health care provider for availability in your area.

Mail-Back Programs

Sharps users place their used sharps in special containers and return the container by mail to a collection site for proper disposal. This service usually

with insulin-dependent diabetes use syringes and lancets every day, but what do you do with them when you're done?

Like anything else we throw out, lancets and syringes need to be disposed of properly. Otherwise they can end up in places they don't belong, like beaches. And because they have very sharp, pointy ends, they can hurt people requires a fee. Fees vary depending on the size of the container. Check with your health care provider, pharmacist, yellow pages, or search the Internet using keywords "sharps mail back."

Syringe Exchange Programs (SEP)

Sharps users can safely exchange used needles for new needles. Contact the North American Syringe Exchange Network at 253-272-4857 or online at <www.nasen.org>.

At-Home Needle Destruction Devices

Several manufacturers offer products that allow you to destroy used needles at home. These devices sever, burn, or melt the needle, rendering it safe for disposal. Check with your pharmacist or search the Internet using keywords "sharps disposal devices." The prices of these devices vary according to product type and manufacturer.

For More Information

- Call your local solid waste department or public health department to determine the correct disposal method for your area.
- Ask your health care provider or local pharmacist if they offer disposal, or if they know of safe disposal programs in the area.
- Contact the Coalition for Safe Community Needle Disposal at 1-800-643-1643. Ask about the availability of safe disposal programs in your area or information on setting up a community disposal program. Visit www.epa.gov/epaoswer/other/medical.

by accident, like the person who collects your garbage, someone in your family, or even you. But there's a simple way you can help protect people and the environment. It's quick and easy.

After you've given yourself an insulin shot, put your syringe directly into a strong plastic or metal container with a tight cap or lid. Don't try to bend, break, or put the cap back on your needle. You might hurt yourself. After you use a lancet, you can put it into the same container too. Keep your container in the same room you usually have your insulin shot or test your blood sugar.

♣ It's A Fact!!
Container Dos

The best containers to use are those that:

- Are made of strong plastic, so needles can't poke through.
- Have a small opening on top with a cap or lid that screws on tightly to prevent spills.
- Are not recyclable in your community. Put recyclable containers back into use whenever possible.

Some examples might include a plastic bleach jug, plastic liquid detergent bottle, or plastic milk jug. You can use a coffee can, too. But when it gets full, close the lid tightly and seal it with strong tape.

Container Don'ts

- Don't use glass containers (they can break), or lightweight plastic containers.
- Don't use any container that will be returned to a store.
- If you use a recyclable container to dispose of syringes and lancets, be sure it doesn't end up in the recycling bin by mistake. These items are not recyclable and could affect the safe and effective recycling of other items in the bin.

When the container is full, tightly secure the lid and reinforce it with heavy-duty tape before throwing it in the trash.

Chapter 23

Insulin Pumps

If you're ready for one, an insulin pump can change your life for the better. Insulin pumps deliver more than insulin. Many people who use them say that pumps also deliver more freedom.

Pumps provide you with a small amount of insulin throughout the day (the basal rate) to keep your blood glucose stable. When you eat, you simply press a button or two, and voila, you've given yourself a bolus, a dose of insulin to handle your food. With a pump, you're not tied to a rigid meal schedule, and you have more flexibility regarding your diet.

The pump can also help you achieve better control over your diabetes, which lowers your risk of developing complications and makes you feel better. Most people who use an insulin pump say they love it.

However, there are responsibilities that come with using an insulin pump. Knowing what they are ahead of time can help you make a smooth transition.

It Requires Education

The pump will be attached to your body through an infusion set. You'll have to learn how to change the infusion set, how to program the pump, and what to do if the infusion set becomes clogged or knocked loose.

About This Chapter: "5 Things You Should Know Before Pumping," by Terri Kordella. Copyright © 2004 American Diabetes Association. From *Diabetes Forecast*, May 2004. Reprinted with permission from The American Diabetes Association.

✎ **What's It Mean?**

Basal Rate: A steady trickle of low levels of longer-acting insulin. [1]

Bolus: An extra amount of insulin taken to cover an expected rise in blood glucose, often related to a meal or snack. [1]

C-Peptide: (Connecting Peptide) A substance the pancreas releases into the bloodstream in equal amounts to insulin. A test of C-peptide levels shows how much insulin the body is making. [1]

Infusion: A method of putting fluids, including drugs, into the bloodstream. Also called intravenous infusion. [2]

Source: [1] "Diabetes Dictionary," National Diabetes Information Clearing-house (NDIC), a publication of the National Institute of Diabetes and Digestive and Kidney Diseases (NIDDK), National Institutes of Health (NIH), NIH Publication No. 04-3016, November 2003; available at http://diabetes.niddk.nih.gov/dm/pubs/dictionary. [2] "Dictionary of Cancer Terms," National Cancer Institute, cited September 2005; available at http://www.cancer.gov.

"It's important to understand the mechanics of the pump and how to choose an appropriate site on your body for inserting the infusion set," says Kristi Shaver, RN, BS, CDE, education coordinator, diabetes nurse educa-tor, and pump trainer at the Joslin Diabetes Center in Syracuse, NY. "If your pump gets clogged, or you have bad absorption, within three or four hours, your blood glucose can run into the 600s, and you can get into trouble pretty quickly."

Clogs (occlusions) are not common, but when they do occur, it's often because the infusion set has been left in the same site for too long. Knowing how to change your infusion set and how often to change it can minimize the risk of clogs in your pump and the resulting high blood glucose.

"Pump education programs are quite thorough and are designed to help you minimize the risk of such problems," says Carolyn M. Grubb, MA, CDE, RD, LD, nutrition consultant and diabetes educator in Austin, Tex.

"Usually, you'll meet with a pump trainer for three or four hours, watch a video, and walk through the steps of programming the pump together," she says. "There might be a checklist for every little thing you have to learn. You might have to take carb-counting classes. You'll need to learn how to balance your insulin with the food you eat and how much you exercise."

"Dietary education is huge," Shaver adds. "You'll need to meet with a dietitian and work out a meal plan, whether it's carb-counting or another consistent way of measuring your intake."

You'll Still Need Back-Up Equipment

"The best-made plans can go awry, however, and pumps are not foolproof," says Nancy Leggett-Frazier, MSN, RN, CDE, diabetes nurse educator at the East Carolina University Brody School of Medicine and adjunct instructor at the Eastern Carolina University School of Nursing in Greenville, NC. "You'll need to carry extra supplies with you in case the infusion set gets clogged or the battery dies. Plus, you'll need syringes, back-up insulin, and all of the other stuff that you already take with you to care for your diabetes."

You'll Still Have To Check Your Blood Glucose

"If you're not willing to check your blood glucose at least four times a day, you won't have a lot of success with a pump," says Leggett-Frazier. "Part of the deal with a pump is that when your blood glucose is not on target, you can make little corrections. You have to check your blood glucose often to see whether you need to correct them."

"The pump is not an artificial pancreas," adds Grubb. "Sometimes people talk as though it is, but it doesn't monitor your blood glucose. You're still going to have to measure your blood glucose levels before you take a bolus and keep tabs on your basal rate."

Also, many insurance companies require 30 to 60 days of records documenting that you check your blood glucose before they offer coverage.

It's Not Cheap

Medicare covers insulin pumps and supplies for people with diabetes (both type 1 and type 2) who meet certain eligibility requirements, including those regarding fasting C-peptide levels. If you have private insurance, coverage is determined by your carrier.

"Most insurance companies pay for about 80 percent of the cost of a pump and pump supplies, but a pump may cost as much as $6,000," says Leggett-Frazier. A 20 percent copayment on a $6,000 pump would be $1,200. Pump supplies can run anywhere from $60 to $80 a month, and you'll probably have to pay a portion of that out of pocket.

"Know ahead of time what your plan covers," says Grubb. "Sometimes there are unpleasant surprises."

It Takes Patience At First

The pump takes some getting used to, even after you've received the appropriate training.

"Even though you can learn how to push the buttons in a few hours, it really takes a few months to get used to using a pump," says Leggett-Frazier. "It's a matter of how your body reacts to the insulin."

Shaver agrees. "When you start using a pump, your basal rate and bolus doses are guesstimates," she says. "You learn by trying different things, and you go by experience."

When you get an insulin pump, the manufacturer will send you plenty of information. Keep all of this information together so you can refer to it quickly and easily. All of the pump companies have toll-free numbers you can call with questions about your pump, and their hotlines are answered by experts who can help you troubleshoot.

But It's Worth It

Once you get the hang of using a pump, chances are your blood glucose control will improve. Better control means a lower risk of developing complications like heart disease, kidney disease, nerve damage, and eye disease. Your quality of life will improve, too.

Grubb sums it up: "The benefits of using a pump far outweigh the time and effort it takes to maintain it. You might be surprised at the benefits, and how much better you'll feel."

♣ It's A Fact!!

Because of the need for fine-tuning, most diabetes centers require that you stay in close contact with your doctor or diabetes educator when you begin using a pump. You should arrange for a way to contact your health care provider as often as you need to at the beginning, as you might need to call him or her as often as once a day for the first week.

Chapter 24

The Future Of Insulin

There are 17 million people in the United States who have diabetes. More than a fifth of them take at least one insulin injection a day. Insulin injections are often necessary for controlling blood sugars to decrease the risk of complications and improve health. For those with type 1 diabetes, it's a matter of day-to-day survival. But type of diabetes aside, insulin shots are a fact of life for almost four million Americans.

For now.

Several companies are working on developing new ways of taking insulin, from pills to patches to mouth sprays to inhalers. Headlines in the popular press may make it seem like these products will be available soon, but the truth is that there is no guarantee that any of them will pass muster. The ones that are furthest along in development are probably years away from becoming available, even if the Food and Drug Administration (FDA) approves them. The exception would be if the FDA decides to "fast-track" any of them. When a product is "fast-tracked," it has priority review, and the FDA may render a decision about approval in as little as six months. That said, several new forms of insulin delivery do look promising. What could be in store? What might the future of insulin look like?

Insulin Inhalers

More companies are working on insulin inhalers than any other insulin delivery option. Insulin inhalers would work much like asthma inhalers. You would breathe the insulin in through your mouth and it would be absorbed through your lungs. The insulin, either a powder or liquid, would be fast acting, so you would take it at mealtime.

There are two challenges with insulin inhalers, however, the rate of absorbency and side effects. Your age and your respiratory shape may affect how much insulin you actually absorb through your lungs. Side effects range from mild cough to more serious, if rare, conditions such as scarring in the lungs.

The front-runner in the race for inhalable insulin appears to be Exubera, a combined effort of Inhale Therapeutic Systems, Inc., Pfizer, Inc., and Aventis Pharma. [Note: For updated information about Exubera, see the note at the end of this chapter.]

Mouth Sprays

Mouth sprays deliver insulin through an aerosol spray. They differ from inhalers, however, because the insulin would be absorbed through the inside of your cheeks and in the back of your mouth instead of your lungs.

Two forms of mouth spray are in development, one that is fast acting and one that would cover the basal rate of insulin. (The basal rate is the amount of insulin you need throughout the day to keep blood sugars stable.) Generex Biotechnology is developing these sprays in Canada and is partnering with Eli Lilly and Company in the United States.

Pills

The biggest challenge with insulin pills to date has been posed by the human digestive system. Either the gastrointestinal tract breaks the insulin down or the insulin passes through the system intact because it is unable to pass through the gastrointestinal membrane. In both situations, the insulin does not make it to the liver and then the bloodstream, which is where it needs to go to reach the muscle cells and do its biochemical duty.

Several manufacturers are working on pills. In these pills, special molecules attached to the insulin would help it reach its destination either by helping to prevent the insulin from being broken down, escorting the insulin through the gastrointestinal lining, or both.

Insulin from pills would reach its peak action about 15 minutes after you swallow them, so pills would be considered fast acting.

The Patch

Most of the other forms of insulin in development are fast acting, so your mealtime dose would be covered. But where does that leave you for basal insulin?

The answer may be an insulin patch from the Altea Development Corporation. Using the patch would be a two-step process. First you would use a device that would make microscopic holes in the top layer of your skin. Then you would apply the patch. Altea is working on a 24-hour patch that you would only have to apply once a day.

The Long Road To Approval

Different methods of insulin delivery are in different stages of development. Each product must go through clinical trials before the company submits an application to the Food and Drug Administration (FDA) for approval.

Pre-Clinical Testing. This is the first consideration of a new product. The company evaluates how a given substance works in test tubes and in laboratory animals. It takes from three to three and a half years for most companies to decide whether to pursue further testing.

Investigational New Drug Application (IND Application). After the company determines that pre-clinical testing was successful, it will file an IND application with the FDA. Then clinical trials may begin.

Phase I. This phase determines the safety and dosage of the substance. There are usually between 20 and 80 healthy volunteers in the trial that do not have the condition the product is meant to treat. Phase I trials last one year.

Phase II. The second phase of clinical trials involves 100 to 300 volunteers who have the condition the product is meant to treat. Researchers evaluate the product's effectiveness and look for side effects. This phase lasts about two years.

Phase III. In the third phase, researchers evaluate the effectiveness of the drug in 1,000 to 3,000 volunteers who have the condition the product is meant to treat. This phase takes about three years and gives researchers a chance to see if there are any adverse effects from long-term use.

New Drug Application (ND Application). If the company is satisfied that the product is safe and effective, it will file a ND application with the FDA to request FDA approval to sell the drug in the United States. FDA review may take as long as two to two and a half years unless the product is fast-tracked.

Phase IV. The final phase, required by the FDA, is also called the "post-marketing" phase. In this phase, the company tracks the product once it is out on the market.

♣ **It's A Fact!!**
In general, for every 5,000 substances drug companies consider, only about five actually enter clinical trials. Of those five, the FDA will approve only one.

Note

On January 27, 2006, the U.S. Food and Drug Administration approved Exubera, an inhaled powder form of recombinant human insulin (rDNA) for the treatment of adult patients with type 1 and type 2 diabetes. The approval marked the first new insulin delivery option introduced since the disovery of insulin in the 1920s. For more information, visit http://www.fda.gov/bbs/topics/news/2006/NEW103004.html.

Chapter 25

Pancreatic Islet Transplantation

The pancreas, an organ about the size of a hand, is located behind the lower part of the stomach. It makes insulin and enzymes that help the body digest and use food. Spread all over the pancreas are clusters of cells called the islets of Langerhans. Islets are made up of two types of cells: alpha cells, which make glucagon, a hormone that raises the level of glucose (sugar) in the blood, and beta cells, which make insulin.

Islet Functions

Insulin is a hormone that helps the body use glucose for energy. If your beta cells do not produce enough insulin, diabetes will develop. In type 1 diabetes, the insulin shortage is caused by an autoimmune process in which the body's immune system destroys the beta cells.

Islet Transplantation

In an experimental procedure called islet transplantation, islets are taken from a donor pancreas and transferred into another person. Once implanted, the beta cells in these islets begin to make and release insulin.

About This Chapter: Excerpted from "Pancreatic Islet Transplantation," a publication of the National Diabetes Information Clearinghouse (NDIC), a service of the National Institute of Diabetes and Digestive and Kidney Diseases (NIDDK), National Institutes of Health (NIH), NIH Publication No. 04-4693, November 2003.

Research Developments

Scientists have made many advances in islet transplantation in recent years. Since reporting their findings in the June 2000 issue of the *New England Journal of Medicine*, researchers at the University of Alberta in Edmonton, Canada, have continued to use a procedure called the Edmonton protocol to transplant pancreatic islets into people with type 1 diabetes. A multicenter clinical trial of the Edmonton protocol for islet transplantation is currently under way, and results will be announced in several years. According to the Immune Tolerance Network (ITN), as of June 2003, about 50 percent of the patients have remained insulin-free up to 1 year after receiving a transplant. A clinical trial of the Edmonton protocol is also being conducted by the ITN funded by the National Institutes of Health and the Juvenile Diabetes Research Foundation International.

Researchers use specialized enzymes to remove islets from the pancreas of a deceased donor. Because the islets are fragile, transplantation occurs soon after they are removed.

During the transplant, the surgeon uses ultrasound to guide placement of a small plastic tube (catheter) through the upper abdomen and into the liver. The islets are then injected through the catheter into the liver. The patient will receive a local anesthetic. If a patient cannot tolerate local anesthesia, the surgeon may use general anesthesia and do the transplant through a small incision. Possible risks include bleeding or blood clots.

It takes time for the cells to attach to new blood vessels and begin releasing insulin. The doctor will order many tests to check blood glucose levels after the transplant, and insulin may be needed until control is achieved.

Transplantation Benefits, Risks, and Obstacles

The goal of islet transplantation is to infuse enough islets to control the blood glucose level without insulin injections. For an average-size person (70 kg), a typical transplant requires about 1 million islets, extracted from two donor pancreases. Because good control of blood glucose can slow or prevent the progression of complications associated with diabetes, such as nerve or eye damage, a successful transplant may reduce the risk of these complications. But a transplant recipient will need to take immunosuppressive drugs that stop the immune system from rejecting the transplanted islets.

Researchers are trying to find new approaches that will allow successful transplantation without the use of immunosuppressive drugs, thus eliminating the side effects that may accompany their long-term use.

♣ It's A Fact!!
Researchers hope that islet transplantation will help people with type 1 diabetes live without daily injections of insulin.

Rejection is the biggest problem with any transplant. The immune system is programmed to destroy bacteria, viruses, and tissue it recognizes as "foreign," including transplanted islets. Immunosuppressive drugs are needed to keep the transplanted islets functioning.

Immunosuppressive Drugs

The Edmonton protocol uses a combination of immunosuppressive drugs, also called antirejection drugs, including dacliximab (Zenapax), sirolimus (Rapamune), and tacrolimus (Prograf). Dacliximab is given intravenously right after the transplant and then discontinued. Sirolimus and tacrolimus, the two main drugs that keep the immune system from destroying the transplanted islets, must be taken for life.

These drugs have significant side effects and their long-term effects are still not known. Immediate side effects of immunosuppressive drugs may include mouth sores and gastrointestinal problems, such as stomach upset or diarrhea. Patients may also have increased blood cholesterol levels, decreased white blood cell counts, decreased kidney function, and increased susceptibility to bacterial and viral infections. Taking immunosuppressive drugs increases the risk of tumors and cancer as well.

Researchers do not fully know what long-term effects this procedure may have. Also, although the early results of the Edmonton protocol are very encouraging, more research is needed to answer questions about how long the islets will survive and how often the transplantation procedure will be successful.

A major obstacle to widespread use of islet transplantation will be the shortage of islet cells. The supply available from deceased donors will be enough for only a small percentage of those with type 1 diabetes. However,

---

♣ It's A Fact!!
Severe Hypoglycemia
Is Rare After Islet Transplantation

Episodes of dangerously low blood glucose, or hypoglycemia, were greatly reduced in people who received an islet transplant for poorly controlled type 1 diabetes, according to an analysis of outcomes in 138 patients who had the procedure at 19 medical centers in the United States and Canada. This is one of the conclusions of the Collaborative Islet Transplant Registry (CITR), which tracks many factors affecting the success of this experimental procedure in people with severe type 1 diabetes.

Nearly all patients receiving a transplant had severe hypoglycemia episodes requiring another person's help before the transplant, but such events are very rare in the year after a successful transplant, the CITR reports. One infusion of islets, though not always enough to keep blood glucose in the normal range, generally lowered insulin needs and alleviated episodes of severely low blood glucose in most patients.

One year after the last infusion, 58 percent of recipients no longer had to inject insulin. Those who still needed insulin a year after their last infusion had a 69 percent reduction in insulin requirements. However, in 19 recipients followed by the registry, the donor islets failed to function. Transplant failures, as measured by blood glucose levels and confirmed by a test of C-peptide, occurred as early as 30 days after the recipient's first islet infusion to more than 2 years after the last infusion.

researchers are pursuing avenues for alternative sources, such as creating islet cells from other types of cells. New technologies could then be employed to grow islet cells in the laboratory.

Eighteen of the 19 centers contributed data on adverse events, including 77 serious adverse events. About 58 percent of the serious events required inpatient hospitalization, and 22 percent were considered life threatening. Seventeen percent of the serious events were linked to the islet infusion procedure (e.g., infection or bleeding), and 27 percent were related to medications that suppress the immune system (e.g., anemia, nerve damage, and low numbers of white blood cells). Recipients received immunosuppressive drugs that usually included Daclizumab at the beginning of the procedure to prevent immune rejection of donor islets, then sirolimus and tacrolimus to maintain immunosuppression.

Recipients had type 1 diabetes an average of 29 years before the transplant. Most—118—received an islet transplant alone. An additional 19 patients had an islet transplant after receiving a kidney transplant. One patient received an autograft transplant of his own islets that were extracted after pancreatic surgery and then infused into the liver. Forty patients received one islet infusion, 69 received two, and 28 received three. A single patient received four infusions.

Recipients, 66 percent of whom were women, were an average age of 42 years (range 24 to 64 years). Their average weight was in the healthy range. Before the procedure, nearly half the recipients were using an insulin pump. Their average level of hemoglobin A1c (HbA1c), which reflects blood glucose control over the previous 3 months, was 7.6 percent, compared to a normal HbA1c of 6 percent. HbA1c levels generally improved with each infusion, as did levels of C-peptide, a measure of insulin secretion.

Part Three
Diabetes And Related Health Concerns

Chapter 26

Hypoglycemia

Hypoglycemia, also called low blood sugar, occurs when your blood glucose (blood sugar) level drops too low to provide enough energy for your body's activities. In adults or children older than 10 years, hypoglycemia is uncommon except as a side effect of diabetes treatment, but it can result from other medications or diseases, hormone or enzyme deficiencies, or tumors.

Glucose, a form of sugar, is an important fuel for your body. Carbohydrates are the main dietary sources of glucose. Rice, potatoes, bread, tortillas, cereal, milk, fruit, and sweets are all carbohydrate-rich foods.

After a meal, glucose molecules are absorbed into your bloodstream and carried to the cells, where they are used for energy. Insulin, a hormone produced by your pancreas, helps glucose enter cells. If you take in more glucose than your body needs at the time, your body stores the extra glucose in your liver and muscles in a form called glycogen. Your body can use the stored glucose whenever it is needed for energy between meals. Extra glucose can also be converted to fat and stored in fat cells.

About This Chapter: Excerpted from "Hypoglycemia," a publication of the National Diabetes Information Clearinghouse (NDIC), a service of the National Institute of Diabetes and Digestive and Kidney Diseases (NIDDK), National Institutes of Health (NIH), NIH Publication No. 03-3926, March 2003.

When blood glucose begins to fall, glucagon, another hormone produced by the pancreas, signals the liver to break down glycogen and release glucose, causing blood glucose levels to rise toward a normal level. If you have diabetes, this glucagon response to hypoglycemia may be impaired, making it harder for your glucose levels to return to the normal range.

Symptoms

Symptoms of hypoglycemia include the following.

- hunger

- nervousness and shakiness

- perspiration

- dizziness or light-headedness

- sleepiness

- confusion

- difficulty speaking

- feeling anxious or weak

Hypoglycemia can also happen while you are sleeping. You might experience things like these:

- cry out or have nightmares

- find that your pajamas or sheets are damp from perspiration

- feel tired, irritable, or confused when you wake up

✎ What's It Mean?

Carbohydrate: One of the three main nutrients in food. Foods that provide carbohydrate are starches, vegetables, fruits, dairy products, and sugars.

Enzyme: Protein made by the body that brings about a chemical reaction, for example, the enzymes produced by the gut to aid digestion.

Glucagon: A hormone produced by the alpha cells in the pancreas. It raises blood glucose. An injectable form of glucagon, available by prescription, may be used to treat severe hypoglycemia.

Hormone: A chemical produced in one part of the body and released into the blood to trigger or regulate particular functions of the body. For example, insulin is a hormone made in the pancreas that tells other cells when to use glucose for energy. Synthetic hormones, made for use as medicines, can be the same or different from those made in the body.

Source: "Diabetes Dictionary," National Diabetes Information Clearinghouse (NDIC), a publication of the National Institute of Diabetes and Digestive and Kidney Diseases (NIDDK), National Institutes of Health (NIH), NIH Publication No. 06-3016, October 2005; available at http://diabetes.niddk.nih.gov/dm/pubs/dictionary.

Hypoglycemia: A Side Effect Of Diabetes Medications

Hypoglycemia can occur in people with diabetes who take certain medications to keep their blood glucose levels in control. Usually hypoglycemia is mild and can easily be treated by eating or drinking something with carbohydrate. But left untreated, hypoglycemia can lead to loss of consciousness. Although hypoglycemia can happen suddenly, it can usually be treated quickly, bringing your blood glucose level back to normal.

Causes Of Hypoglycemia

In people taking certain blood-glucose lowering medications, blood glucose can fall too low for a number of reasons:

- Meals or snacks that are too small, delayed, or skipped

- Excessive doses of insulin or some diabetes medications, including sulfonylureas and meglitinides (Alpha-glucosidase inhibitors, biguanides, and thiazolidinediones alone should not cause hypoglycemia but can when used with other diabetes medicines.)

- Increased activity or exercise

- Excessive drinking of alcohol

Prevention

Your diabetes treatment plan is designed to match your medication dosage and schedule to your usual meals and activities. If you take insulin but then skip a meal, the insulin will still lower your blood glucose, but it will not find the food it is designed to break down. This mismatch might result in hypoglycemia.

To help prevent hypoglycemia, you should keep in mind several things:

- **Your diabetes medications.** Some medications can cause hypoglycemia. Ask your health care provider if yours can. Also, always take medications and insulin in the recommended doses and at the recommended times.

- **Your meal plan.** Meet with a registered dietitian and agree on a meal plan that fits your preferences and lifestyle. Do your best to follow this meal plan most of the time. Eat regular meals, have enough food at each meal, and try not to skip meals or snacks.

- **Your daily activity.** Talk to your health care team about whether you should have a snack or adjust your medication before sports or exercise. If you know that you will be more active than usual or will be doing something that is not part of your normal routine, shoveling snow for example, consider having a snack first.

✔ Quick Tip

What To Ask Your Doctor About Your Diabetes Medications

- Could my diabetes medication cause hypoglycemia?

- When should I take my diabetes medication?

- How much should I take?

- Should I keep taking my diabetes medication if I am sick?

- Should I adjust my medication before exercise?

- **Alcoholic beverages.** Drinking, especially on an empty stomach, can cause hypoglycemia, even a day or two later. People who drink an alcoholic beverage, should always have a snack or meal at the same time.

- **Your diabetes management plan.** Intensive diabetes management—keeping your blood glucose as close to the normal range as possible to prevent long-term complications—can increase the risk of hypoglycemia. If your goal is tight control, talk to your health care team about ways to prevent hypoglycemia and how best to treat it if it does occur.

Treatment

If you think your blood glucose is too low, use a blood glucose meter to check your level. If it is 70 mg/dL or below, have one of these "quick fix" foods right away to raise your blood glucose:

- 2 or 3 glucose tablets

- ½ cup (4 ounces) of any fruit juice

- ½ cup (4 ounces) of a regular (not diet) soft drink

- 1 cup (8 ounces) of milk

- 5 or 6 pieces of hard candy

- 1 or 2 teaspoons of sugar or honey

After 15 minutes, check your blood glucose again to make sure that it is no longer too low. If it is still too low, have another serving. Repeat these steps until your blood glucose is at least 70. Then, if it will be an hour or more before your next meal, have a snack.

If you take insulin or a diabetes medication that can cause hypoglycemia, always carry one of the quick-fix foods with you. Wearing a medical identification bracelet or necklace is also a good idea.

Exercise can also cause hypoglycemia. Check your blood glucose before you exercise.

Severe hypoglycemia can cause you to lose consciousness. In these extreme cases when you lose consciousness and cannot eat, glucagon can be injected to quickly raise your blood glucose level. Ask your health care provider if having a glucagon kit at home and at work is appropriate for you. This is particularly important if you have type 1 diabetes. Your family, friends, and coworkers will need to be taught how to give you a glucagon injection in an emergency.

Prevention of hypoglycemia while you are driving a vehicle is especially important. Checking blood glucose frequently and snacking as needed to keep your blood glucose above 70 mg/dL will help prevent accidents.

Hypoglycemia In People Who Do Not Have Diabetes

Two types of hypoglycemia can occur in people who do not have diabetes: reactive (postprandial, or after meals) and fasting (postabsorptive). Reactive hypoglycemia is not usually related to any underlying disease; fasting hypoglycemia often is.

Symptoms

Symptoms of both types resemble the symptoms that people with diabetes and hypoglycemia experience: hunger, nervousness, perspiration, shakiness, dizziness, light-headedness, sleepiness, confusion, difficulty speaking, and feeling anxious or weak.

If you are diagnosed with hypoglycemia, your doctor will try to find the cause by using laboratory tests to measure blood glucose, insulin, and other chemicals that play a part in the body's use of energy.

✔ **Quick Tip**
Signs and symptoms of hypoglycemia can vary from person to person. Get to know your own signs and describe them to your friends and family so they will be able to help you.

If you experience hypoglycemia several times a week, call your health care provider. You may need a change in your treatment plan: less medication or a different medication, a new schedule for your insulin shots or medication, a different meal plan, or a new exercise plan.

Reactive Hypoglycemia

In reactive hypoglycemia, symptoms appear within 4 hours after you eat a meal.

Diagnosis: To diagnose reactive hypoglycemia, your doctor may:

• ask you about signs and symptoms.

• test your blood glucose while you are having symptoms. (The doctor will take a blood sample from your arm and send it to a laboratory for analysis. A personal blood glucose monitor cannot be used to diagnose reactive hypoglycemia.)

• check to see whether your symptoms ease after your blood glucose returns to 70 or above (after eating or drinking).

A blood glucose level of less than 70 mg/dL at the time of symptoms and relief after eating will confirm the diagnosis.

The oral glucose tolerance test is no longer used to diagnose hypoglycemia; experts now know that the test can actually trigger hypoglycemic symptoms.

Causes And Treatment: The causes of most cases of reactive hypoglycemia are still open to debate. Some researchers suggest that certain people may be more sensitive to the body's normal release of the hormone epinephrine, which causes many of the symptoms of hypoglycemia. Others believe that deficiencies in glucagon secretion might lead to hypoglycemia.

A few causes of reactive hypoglycemia are certain, but they are uncommon. Gastric (stomach) surgery, for instance, can cause hypoglycemia because of the rapid passage of food into the small intestine. Also, rare enzyme deficiencies diagnosed early in life, such as hereditary fructose intolerance, may cause reactive hypoglycemia.

To relieve reactive hypoglycemia, some health professionals recommend taking the following steps:

- Eat small meals and snacks about every 3 hours.

- Exercise regularly.

- Eat a variety of foods, including meat, poultry, fish, or non-meat sources of protein; starchy foods such as whole-grain bread, rice, and potatoes; fruits; vegetables; and dairy products.

- Choose high-fiber foods.

- Avoid or limit foods high in sugar, especially on an empty stomach.

Your doctor can refer you to a registered dietitian for personalized meal-planning advice. Although some health professionals recommend a diet high in protein and low in carbohydrates, studies have not proven the effectiveness of this kind of diet for reactive hypoglycemia.

Fasting Hypoglycemia

Diagnosis: Fasting hypoglycemia is diagnosed from a blood sample that shows a blood glucose level of less than 50 mg/dL after an overnight fast, between meals, or after exercise.

Causes And Treatment: Causes include certain medications, alcohol, critical illnesses, hormonal deficiencies, some kinds of tumors, and certain conditions occurring in infancy and childhood.

Medications: Medications, including some used to treat diabetes, are the most common cause of hypoglycemia. Other medications that can cause hypoglycemia include:

- salicylates, including aspirin, when taken in large doses.
- sulfa medicines, which are used to treat infections.
- pentamidine, which treats a very serious kind of pneumonia.
- quinine, which is used to treat malaria.

If using any of these medications causes your blood glucose to drop, your doctor may advise you to stop using the drug or change the dosage.

Alcohol: Drinking, especially binge drinking, can cause hypoglycemia because your body's breakdown of alcohol interferes with your liver's efforts to raise blood glucose. Hypoglycemia caused by excessive drinking can be very serious and even fatal.

Critical Illnesses: Some illnesses that affect the liver, heart, or kidneys can cause hypoglycemia. Sepsis (overwhelming infection) and starvation are other causes of hypoglycemia. In these cases, treatment targets the underlying cause.

Hormonal Deficiencies: Hormonal deficiencies may cause hypoglycemia in very young children, but usually not in adults. Shortages of cortisol, growth hormone, glucagon, or epinephrine can lead to fasting hypoglycemia. Laboratory tests for hormone levels will determine a diagnosis and treatment. Hormone replacement therapy may be advised.

Tumors: Insulinomas, insulin-producing tumors, can cause hypoglycemia by raising your insulin levels too high in relation to your blood glucose level. These tumors are very rare and do not normally spread to other parts of the body. Laboratory tests can pinpoint the exact cause. Treatment involves both short-term steps to correct the hypoglycemia and medical or surgical measures to remove the tumor.

Conditions Occurring In Infancy And Childhood

Children rarely develop hypoglycemia. If they do, causes may include:

- brief intolerance to fasting, often in conjunction with an illness that disturbs regular eating patterns. Children usually outgrow this tendency by age 10.

- hyperinsulinism, which is the excessive production of insulin. This condition can result in transient neonatal hypoglycemia, which is common in infants of mothers with diabetes. Persistent hyperinsulinism in infants or children is a complex disorder that requires prompt evaluation and treatment by a specialist.

- enzyme deficiencies that affect carbohydrate metabolism. These deficiencies can interfere with the body's ability to process natural sugars, such as fructose and galactose, glycogen, or other metabolites.

- hormonal deficiencies such as lack of pituitary or adrenal hormones.

Chapter 27

Hyperglycemia

What is a high blood glucose?

People who do not have diabetes typically have fasting plasma blood glucose levels that run under 126 mg/dl.

Your physician will define for you what your target blood glucose should be—identifying a blood glucose target that is as close to normal as possible that you can safely achieve given your overall medical health. In general, high blood glucose, also called hyperglycemia, is considered high when it is 160 mg/dl or above your individual blood glucose target. Be sure to ask your health care provider what he or she thinks is a safe target for you for blood glucose before and after meals. If your blood glucose runs high for long periods of time, this can pose significant problems for you long-term—increased risk of complications, such as eye disease, kidney disease, heart attacks and strokes and more. High blood glucose can pose health problems in the short-term as well. Your treatment plan may need adjustment if the blood glucose stays over 180 mg/dl for 3 days in a row.

What are the symptoms of high blood glucose?

- Increased thirst

- Increased urination

- Dry mouth or skin

- Tiredness or fatigue

- Blurred vision

- More frequent infections

- Slow healing cuts and sores

- Unexplained weight loss

What causes a high blood glucose?

- Too much food

- Too little exercise or physical activity

- Not enough diabetes pills or insulin

- "Bad" or spoiled insulin

- Illness, infection, injury, or surgery

- A blood glucose meter that is not reading accurately

✎ What's It Mean?

Ketones: A chemical produced when there is a shortage of insulin in the blood and the body breaks down body fat for energy. High levels of ketones can lead to diabetic ketoacidosis and coma. Sometimes referred to as ketone bodies.

Source: "Diabetes Dictionary," National Diabetes Information Clearinghouse (NDIC), a publication of the National Institute of Diabetes and Digestive and Kidney Diseases (NIDDK), National Institutes of Health (NIH), NIH Publication No. 04-3016, November 2003; available at http://diabetes.niddk.nih.gov/dm/pubs/dictionary.

What should you do for high blood glucose?

1. Be sure to drink plenty of water. It is recommended to drink a minimum of 8 glasses each day.

2. If your blood glucose is 250 or greater and you are on insulin, check your urine for ketones. If you have ketones, follow your sick day rules or call your health care team if you are not sure what to do.

3. Ask yourself what may have caused the high blood sugar, and take action to correct it. Ask your health care team if you are not sure what to do.

4. Try to determine if there is a pattern to your blood glucose levels. Check your blood glucose before meals 3 days in a row.

   • If greater than your target level for 3 days, a change in medication may be needed.

   • Call your health care team or adjust your insulin dose following well day rules.

   • Call your health care team if you are currently using diabetes pills.

🖝 Remember!!

It is important to aim to keep your blood glucose under control, and treat hyperglycemia when it occurs.

Chapter 28

Eye Problems Caused By Diabetes

What can I do to prevent diabetes eye problems?

- Keep your blood glucose and blood pressure as close to normal as you can.

- Have an eye doctor examine your eyes once a year. Have this exam even if your vision is OK. The eye doctor will use drops to make the black part of your eyes (pupils) bigger. This is called dilating (DY-lay-ting) your pupil, which allows the doctor to see the back of your eye. Finding eye problems early and getting treatment right away will help prevent more serious problems later on.

- Ask your eye doctor to check for signs of cataracts and glaucoma. (See "Does diabetes cause other eye problems?" to learn more about cataracts and glaucoma.)

- If you are pregnant and have diabetes, see an eye doctor during your first 3 months.

- If you are planning to get pregnant, ask your doctor if you should have an eye exam.

- Don't smoke.

About This Chapter: Excerpted from "Prevent Diabetes Problems: Keep Your Eyes Healthy," a publication of the National Diabetes Information Clearinghouse (NDIC), a service of the National Institute of Diabetes and Digestive and Kidney Diseases (NIDDK), National Institutes of Health (NIH), NIH Publication No. 04-4279, February 2004.

How can diabetes hurt my eyes?

High blood glucose and high blood pressure from diabetes can hurt four parts of your eye:

1. **Retina** (REH-ti-nuh). The retina is the lining at the back of the eye. The retina's job is to sense light coming into the eye.

2. **Vitreous** (VIH-tree-us). The vitreous is a jelly-like fluid that fills the back of the eye.

3. **Lens.** The lens is at the front of the eye and it focuses light on the retina.

4. **Optic nerve.** The optic nerve is the eye's main nerve to the brain.

How can diabetes hurt the retinas of my eyes?

Retina damage happens slowly. Your retinas have tiny blood vessels that are easy to damage. Having high blood glucose and high blood pressure for a long time can damage these tiny blood vessels.

First, these tiny blood vessels swell and weaken. Some blood vessels then become clogged and do not let enough blood through. At first, you might not have any loss of sight from these changes. This is why you need to have a dilated eye exam once a year even if your sight seems fine.

One of your eyes may be damaged more than the other. Or both eyes may have the same amount of damage.

Diabetic retinopathy (REH-tih-NOP-uh-thee) is the medical term for the most common diabetes eye problem.

What happens as diabetes retina problems get worse?

As diabetes retina problems get worse, new blood vessels grow. These new blood vessels are weak. They break easily and leak blood into the vitreous of your eye. The leaking blood keeps light from reaching the retina.

You may see floating spots or almost total darkness. Sometimes the blood will clear out by itself. But you might need surgery to remove it.

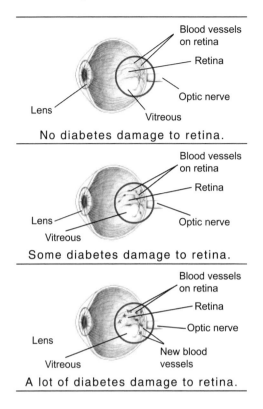

Blood vessels
on retina

Retina

Optic nerve

Lens

Vitreous

No diabetes damage to retina.

Blood vessels
on retina

Retina

Lens

Optic nerve

Vitreous

Some diabetes damage to retina.

Blood vessels
on retina

Retina

Optic nerve

Lens

New blood
vessels

Vitreous

A lot of diabetes damage to retina.

Figure 28.1. Progression of diabetes-related retina problems.

Over the years, the swollen and weak blood vessels can form scar tissue and pull the retina away from the back of the eye. If the retina becomes detached, you may see floating spots or flashing lights.

You may feel as if a curtain has been pulled over part of what you are looking at. A detached retina can cause loss of sight or blindness if you don't take care of it right away.

Call your doctor right away if you are having any vision problems or if you have had a sudden change in your vision.

What can I do about diabetes retina problems?

First, keep your blood glucose and blood pressure as close to normal as you can.

Your eye doctor may suggest laser treatment, which is when a light beam is aimed into the retina of the damaged eye. The beam closes off leaking blood vessels. It may stop blood and fluid from leaking into the vitreous. Laser treatment may slow the loss of sight.

♣ It's A Fact!!
Diabetic Retinopathy Occurs In Pre-Diabetes

Diabetic retinopathy has been found in nearly 8 percent of pre-diabetic participants in the Diabetes Prevention Program (DPP), according to a report presented at the American Diabetes Association's 65th Annual Scientific Sessions. Diabetic retinopathy, which can lead to vision loss, was also seen in 12 percent of participants with type 2 diabetes who developed diabetes during the DPP. No other long-term study has evaluated retinopathy in a population so carefully examined for the presence or development of type 2 diabetes.

"Previous studies have not accurately defined when type 2 diabetes begins, so our understanding of the onset of diabetic eye disease has been limited. Now we know that diabetic retinopathy does occur in pre-diabetes. We're also seeing it early in the course of diabetes—within an average of 3 years after diagnosis," noted Richard Hamman, M.D., DrPH, professor and chair, Department of Preventive Medicine and Biometrics, University of Colorado School of Medicine, and vice chair of the DPP. "This adds to our understanding of the development of retinopathy and suggests that changes in the eye may be starting earlier and at lower glucose levels than we previously thought."

Pre-diabetes is a condition in which blood glucose levels are higher than normal but not high enough for a diagnosis of diabetes. The condition is sometimes called "impaired fasting glucose (IFG)" or "impaired glucose tolerance (IGT)," depending on the test used to diagnose it. People with pre-diabetes have an increased risk of developing type 2 diabetes, heart disease, and stroke.

"Certain retinopathy lesions are considered indicative of the presence of diabetes because they are the first retinal changes to develop in this disease," explained Dr. Hamman. "Although the retinopathy seen in the DPP participants was at a very early stage and did not affect vision, eye changes typical for diabetes were found in 8 percent of our study population before they developed diabetes. These observations may lead diabetes experts to reconsider the

If a lot of blood has leaked into your vitreous and your sight is poor, your eye doctor might suggest you have surgery called a vitrectomy (vih-TREK-tuh-mee). A vitrectomy removes blood and fluids from the vitreous of your eye. Then clean fluid is put back into the eye. The surgery often makes your eyesight better.

diagnostic thresholds used to define diabetes, which are based on levels of blood glucose associated with the development of eye, nerve, and kidney complications of diabetes."

DPP study chair David Nathan, M.D., of Massachusetts General Hospital, pointed out that the retinopathy results are based on a random sample of only 12 percent of DPP participants, all of whom had impaired glucose tolerance, a form of pre-diabetes, when the study began. "These initial findings confirm what other studies have suggested. The complications of diabetes may begin before diabetes is diagnosed, at least by the current-day standards," he explained. "Ideally, an expanded study of the remaining 88 percent of DPP Outcome Study participants might enable us to define more appropriate diagnostic thresholds."

Three hundred two, or about 12 percent, of the DPP Outcome Study participants who had not developed diabetes during the study, and 588 of 876 participants who had developed diabetes, were selected to participate in the retinopathy study, funded by the National Eye Institute (NEI). To detect diabetic retinopathy, an evaluation of the fundus (inner lining of the eye) was performed with a special camera that provides a detailed look at the retina. Small changes in the vessels, called microaneurysms and hemorrhages, signal the development and degree of retinopathy severity.

Participants with pre-diabetes and retinopathy typically had a small number of microaneurysms in the eye characteristic of early, mild retinopathy that is not yet linked to vision loss. Those who had developed diabetes in the previous 1 to 5 years had slightly more severe retinopathy. Higher average blood glucose levels and higher blood pressure were associated with the risk of developing retinopathy in the new-onset diabetic patients, similar to previous findings in people with long-standing diabetes who develop retinopathy.

Source: Excerpted from "Diabetic Retinopathy Occurs in Pre-Diabetes," NIH News, a publication of the National Institutes of Health (NIH), U.S. Department of Health and Human Services, June 2005.

How do I know if I have retina damage from diabetes?

You may not get any signs of diabetes retina damage or you may get one or more signs:

- Blurry or double vision

- Rings, flashing lights, or blank spots

- Dark or floating spots

- Pain or pressure in one or both of your eyes

- Trouble seeing things out of the corners of your eyes

Does diabetes cause other eye problems?

Yes. You can get two other eye problems—cataracts and glaucoma. People without diabetes can get these eye problems, too. But people with diabetes get them more often and at a younger age.

- A **cataract** (KA-ter-act) is a cloud over the lens of your eye, which is usually clear. The lens focuses light onto the retina. A cataract makes everything you look at seem cloudy. You need surgery to remove the cataract. During surgery your lens is taken out and a plastic lens, like a contact lens, is put in. The plastic lens stays in your eye all the time. Cataract surgery helps you see clearly again.

- **Glaucoma** (glaw-KOH-muh) starts from pressure building up in the eye. Over time, this pressure damages your eye's main nerve—the optic nerve. The damage first causes you to lose sight from the sides of your eyes. Treating glaucoma is usually simple. Your eye doctor will give you special drops to use every day to lower the pressure in your eye. Or your eye doctor may want you to have laser surgery.

Chapter 29

Foot And Skin Problems Caused By Diabetes

How can diabetes hurt my feet?

High blood glucose from diabetes causes two problems that can hurt your feet:

1. **Nerve damage.** One problem is damage to nerves in your legs and feet. With damaged nerves, you might not feel pain, heat, or cold in your legs and feet. A sore or cut on your foot may get worse because you do not know it is there. This lack of feeling is caused by nerve damage, also called diabetic neuropathy (ne-ROP-uh-thee). It can lead to a large sore or infection.

2. **Poor blood flow.** The second problem happens when not enough blood flows to your legs and feet. Poor blood flow makes it hard for a sore or infection to heal. This problem is called peripheral (puh-RIF-uh-rul) vascular disease. Smoking when you have diabetes makes blood flow problems much worse.

These two problems can work together to cause a foot problem.

For example, you get a blister from shoes that do not fit. You do not feel the pain from the blister because you have nerve damage in your foot. Next,

About This Chapter: Excerpted from "Prevent Diabetes Problems: Keep Your Feet and Skin Healthy," a publication of the National Diabetes Information Clearinghouse (NDIC), a service of the National Institute of Diabetes and Digestive and Kidney Diseases (NIDDK), National Institutes of Health (NIH), NIH Publication No. 03-4282, September 2003.

the blister gets infected. If blood glucose is high, the extra glucose feeds the germs. Germs grow and the infection gets worse. Poor blood flow to your legs and feet can slow down healing. Once in a while a bad infection never heals. The infection might cause gangrene (GANG-green). If a person has gangrene, the skin and tissue around the sore die. The area becomes black and smelly.

To keep gangrene from spreading, a doctor may have to do surgery to cut off a toe, foot, or part of a leg. Cutting off a body part is called an amputation (amp-yoo-TAY-shun).

What can I do to take care of my feet?

- **Wash your feet in warm water every day.** Make sure the water is not too hot by testing the temperature with your elbow. Do not soak your feet. Dry your feet well, especially between your toes.

- **Look at your feet every day to check for cuts, sores, blisters, redness, calluses, or other problems.** Checking every day is even more important if you have nerve damage or poor blood flow. If you cannot bend over or pull your feet up to check them, use a mirror.

- **If your skin is dry, rub lotion on your feet after you wash and dry them.** Do not put lotion between your toes

- **File corns and calluses gently with an emery board or pumice stone.** Do this after your bath or shower.

- **Cut your toenails once a week or when needed.** Cut toenails when they are soft from washing. Cut them to the shape of the toe and not too short. File the edges with an emery board.

- **Always wear shoes or slippers to protect your feet from injuries.**

- **Always wear socks or stockings to avoid blisters.** Do not wear socks or knee-high stockings that are too tight below your knee.

- **Wear shoes that fit well.** Shop for shoes at the end of the day when your feet are bigger. Break in shoes slowly. Wear them 1 to 2 hours each day for the first 1 to 2 weeks.

- Before putting your shoes on, feel the insides to make sure they have no sharp edges or objects that might injure your feet.

How can I get my doctor to help me take care of my feet?

- Tell your doctor right away about any foot problems.

- Ask your doctor to look at your feet at each diabetes checkup. To make sure your doctor checks your feet, take off your shoes and socks before your doctor comes into the room.

- Ask your doctor to check how well the nerves in your feet sense feeling.

- Ask your doctor to check how well blood is flowing to your legs and feet.

- Ask your doctor to show you the best way to trim your toenails. Ask what lotion or cream to use on your legs and feet.

- If you cannot cut your toenails or you have a foot problem, ask your doctor to send you to a foot doctor. A doctor who cares for feet is called a podiatrist (puh-DY-uh-trist).

What are common diabetes foot problems?

Anyone can have corns, blisters, and athlete's foot. If you have diabetes and your blood glucose stays high, these foot problems can lead to infections.

- **Corns** and **calluses** are thick layers of skin caused by too much rubbing or pressure on the same spot. Corns and calluses can become infected.

- **Blisters** can form if shoes always rub the same spot. Wearing shoes that do not fit or wearing shoes without socks can cause blisters. Blisters can become infected.

- **Ingrown toenails** happen when an edge of the nail grows into the skin. The skin can get red and infected. Ingrown toenails can happen if you cut into the corners of your toenails when you trim them. If toenail edges are sharp, smooth them with an emery board. You can also get an ingrown toenail if your shoes are too tight.

- A **bunion** forms when your big toe slants toward the small toes and the place between the bones near the base of your big toe grows big. This spot can get red, sore, and infected. Bunions can form on one or both feet. Pointy shoes may cause bunions. Bunions often run in the family. Surgery can remove bunions.

- **Plantar warts** are caused by a virus. The warts usually form on the bottoms of the feet.

- **Hammertoes** form when a foot muscle gets weak. The weakness may be from diabetic nerve damage. The weakened muscle makes the tendons in the foot shorter and makes the toes curl under the feet. You may get sores on the bottoms of your feet and on the tops of your toes. The feet can change their shape. Hammertoes can cause problems with walking and finding shoes that fit well. Hammertoes can run in the family. Wearing shoes that are too short can also cause hammertoes.

- **Dry and cracked skin** can happen because the nerves in your legs and feet do not get the message to keep your skin soft and moist. Dry skin can become cracked and allow germs to enter. If your blood glucose is high, it feeds the germs and makes the infection worse.

- **Athlete's foot** is a fungus that causes redness and cracking of the skin. It is itchy. The cracks between the toes allow germs to get under the skin. If your blood glucose is high, it feeds the germs and makes the infection worse. The infection can spread to the toenails and make them thick, yellow, and hard to cut.

All of these foot problems can be taken care of.

Remember!!
Tell your doctor about any foot problem as soon as you see it.

How can special shoes help my feet?

Special shoes can be made to fit softly around your sore feet or feet that have changed shape. These special shoes help protect your feet. Medicare and other health insurance programs may pay for special shoes. Talk to your doctor about how and where to get them.

How can diabetes hurt my skin?

Drinking fluids helps keep your skin moist and healthy.

Diabetes can hurt your skin in two ways:

1. If your blood glucose is high, your body loses fluid. With less fluid in your body, your skin can get dry. Dry skin can be itchy, causing you to scratch and make it sore. Also, dry skin can crack. Cracks allow germs to enter and cause infection. If your blood glucose is high, it feeds germs and makes infections worse. Skin can get dry on your legs, feet, elbows, and other places on your body.

2. Nerve damage can decrease the amount you sweat. Sweating helps keep your skin soft and moist. Decreased sweating in your feet and legs can cause dry skin.

What can I do to take care of my skin?

- After you wash with a mild soap, make sure you rinse and dry yourself well. Check places where water can hide, such as under the arms, under the breasts, between the legs, and between the toes.

- Keep your skin moist by washing with a mild soap and using lotion or cream after you wash.

- Keep your skin moist by using a lotion or cream after you wash. Ask your doctor to suggest one.

- Drink lots of fluids, such as water, to keep your skin moist and healthy.

- Wear all-cotton underwear. Cotton allows air to move around your body better.

- Check your skin after you wash. Make sure you have no dry, red, or sore spots that might lead to an infection.

- Tell your doctor about any skin problems.

Chapter 30

Tooth And Gum Problems Caused By Diabetes

How can diabetes hurt my teeth and gums?

Tooth and gum problems can happen to anyone. A sticky film full of germs (called plaque [PLAK]) builds up on your teeth. High blood glucose helps germs (bacteria) grow. Then you can get red, sore, and swollen gums that bleed when you brush your teeth.

People with diabetes can have tooth and gum problems more often if their blood glucose stays high. High blood glucose can make tooth and gum problems worse. You can even lose your teeth.

Smoking makes it more likely for you to get a bad case of gum disease, especially if you have diabetes and are age 45 or older.

Red, sore, and bleeding gums are the first sign of gum disease. This can lead to periodontitis (PER-ee-oh-don-TY-tis). Periodontitis is an infection in the gums and the bone that holds the teeth in place. If the infection gets worse, your gums may pull away from your teeth, making your teeth look long.

Call your dentist if you think you have problems with your teeth or gums.

About This Chapter: Excerpted from "Prevent Diabetes Problems: Keep Your Teeth and Gums Healthy," a publication of the National Diabetes Information Clearinghouse (NDIC), a service of the National Institute of Diabetes and Digestive and Kidney Diseases (NIDDK), National Institutes of Health (NIH), NIH Publication No. 03-4280, September 2003.

How do I know if I have damage to my teeth and gums?

If you have one or more of these problems, you may have tooth and gum damage from diabetes:

- Red, sore, swollen gums

- Bleeding gums

- Gums pulling away from your teeth so your teeth look long

- Loose or sensitive teeth

- Bad breath

- A bite that feels different

How can I keep my teeth and gums healthy?

- Keep your blood glucose as close to normal as possible.

- Use dental floss at least once a day. Flossing helps prevent the buildup of plaque on your teeth. Plaque can harden and grow under your gums and cause problems. Using a sawing motion, gently bring the floss between the teeth, scraping from bottom to top several times.

- Brush your teeth after each meal and snack. Use a soft toothbrush. Turn the bristles against the gum line and brush gently. Use small, circular motions. Brush the front, back, and top of each tooth.

- Ask the person who cleans your teeth to show you the best way to brush and floss your teeth and gums. Ask this person about the best toothbrush and toothpaste to use.

- Call your dentist right away if you have problems with your teeth and gums.

- Call your dentist if you have red, sore, or bleeding gums; gums that are pulling away from your teeth; a sore tooth that could be infected.

- Get your teeth and gums cleaned and checked by your dentist twice a year.

- If your dentist tells you about a problem, take care of it right away.

- Be sure your dentist knows that you have diabetes.

- If you smoke, talk to your doctor about ways to quit smoking.

How can my dentist take care of my teeth and gums?

Your dentist can help you take care of your teeth and gums by

- cleaning and checking your teeth and gums twice a year.

- helping you learn the best way to brush and floss your teeth and gums.

- telling you if you have problems with your teeth or gums and what to do about them.

Plan ahead. You may be taking a diabetes medicine that can make your blood glucose too low. This very low blood glucose is called hypoglycemia (hy-po-gly-SEE-mee-uh). If so, talk to your doctor and dentist before the visit about the best way to take care of your blood glucose during the dental work. You may need to bring some diabetes medicine and food with you to the dentist's office.

If your mouth is sore after the dental work, you might not be able to eat or chew for several hours or days. For guidance on how to adjust your normal routine while your mouth is healing, ask your doctor

- what foods and drinks you should have.

- how you should change your diabetes medicines.

- how often you should check your blood glucose.

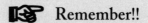 **Remember!!**
Be sure your dentist knows that you have diabetes.

Chapter 31

Kidney Problems Caused By Diabetes

What do my kidneys do?

The kidneys act as filters to clean the blood. They get rid of waste and extra fluid. The tiny filters throughout the kidneys are called glomeruli (gloh-MEHR-yoo-lie).

When kidneys are healthy, the artery (AR-ter-ee) brings blood and waste from the bloodstream into the kidney. The glomeruli clean the blood. Then waste and extra fluid go out into the urine through the ureter. Clean blood goes out of the kidney and back into the bloodstream through the vein.

How can I prevent diabetes kidney problems?

- Keep your blood glucose as close to normal as you can. Ask your doctor what blood glucose numbers are healthy for you.

- Keep your blood pressure below 130/80 to help prevent kidney damage. Blood pressure is written with two numbers separated by a slash. For example: 120/70.

About This Chapter: Excerpted from "Prevent Diabetes Problems: Keep Your Kidneys Healthy," a publication of the National Diabetes Information Clearinghouse (NDIC), a service of the National Institute of Diabetes and Digestive and Kidney Diseases (NIDDK), National Institutes of Health (NIH), NIH Publication No. 03-4281, September 2003.

Ask your doctor what numbers are best for you. If you take blood pressure pills, take them as your doctor tells you. Keeping your blood pressure under control will also slow damage to your eyes, heart, and blood vessels.

- If needed, take blood pressure pills that can also slow down kidney damage. Two kinds of pills can help:
    - ACE (angiotensin [an-gee-oh-TEN-sin] converting enzyme) inhibitor (in-HIB-it-ur)
    - ARB (angiotensin receptor blocker)
- Follow the healthy eating plan you work out with your doctor or dietitian. If you already have kidney problems, your dietitian may suggest that you cut back on protein, such as meat.

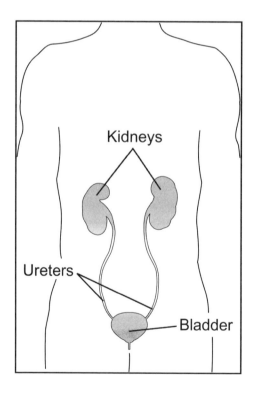

Figure 31.1. High blood glucose can cause kidney problems.

- Have your kidneys checked at least once a year by having your urine tested for small amounts of protein.

- Have any other kidney tests that your doctor thinks you need.

- See a doctor for bladder or kidney infections right away. You may have an infection if you have these symptoms:

    - pain or burning when you urinate

    - frequent urge to go to the bathroom

    - urine that looks cloudy or reddish

    - fever or a shaky feeling

    - pain in your back or on your side below your ribs

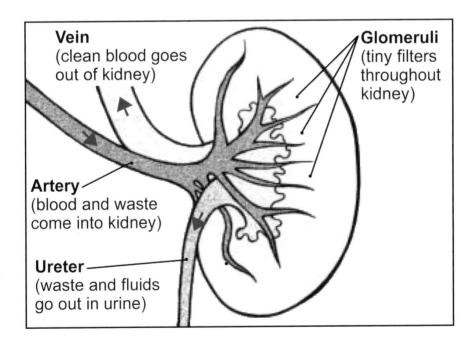

Figure 31.2. You have two kidneys. Your kidneys clean your blood and make urine. Here is a simplified drawing of one.

How can my doctor protect my kidneys during special x-ray tests?

If you have kidney damage, the liquid, called a contrast agent, used for special x-ray tests can make your kidney damage worse. Your doctor can give you extra water before and after the x-ray to protect your kidneys. Or your doctor may decide to order a test that does not use a contrast agent.

How can diabetes hurt my kidneys?

When kidneys are working well, the tiny filters in your kidneys, the glomeruli, keep protein inside your body. You need the protein to stay healthy.

High blood glucose and high blood pressure damage the kidneys' filters. When the kidneys are damaged, the protein leaks out of the kidneys into the urine. Damaged kidneys do not do a good job of cleaning out waste and extra fluids. So not enough waste and fluids go out of the body as urine. Instead, they build up in your blood.

An early sign of kidney damage is when your kidneys leak small amounts of a protein called albumin (al-BYOO-min) into the urine.

With more damage, the kidneys leak more and more protein. This problem is called proteinuria (PRO-tee-NOOR-ee-uh). More and more wastes build up in the blood. This damage gets worse until the kidneys fail.

Diabetic nephropathy (neh-FROP-uh-thee) is the medical term for kidney problems caused by diabetes.

What can I do if I have diabetes kidney problems?

Once you have kidney damage, you cannot undo it. But you can slow it down or stop it from getting worse by doing the same things you would do to prevent kidney problems.

How will I know if my kidneys fail?

At first, you cannot tell. Kidney failure from diabetes happens so slowly that you may not feel sick at all for many years. You will not feel sick even when your kidneys do only half the job of normal kidneys. You may not feel any signs of kidney failure until your kidneys have almost stopped working.

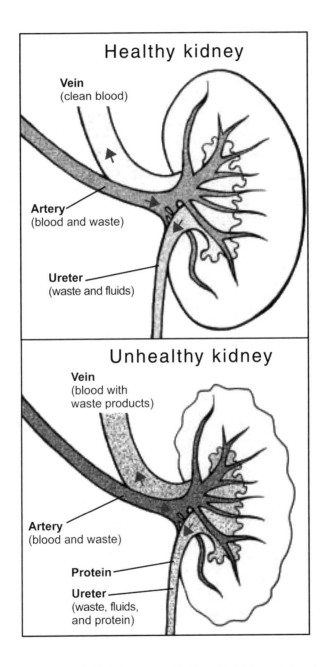

Figure 31.3. No protein is leaking from the healthy kidney (above); protein is leaking from the unhealthy kidney (below).

However, getting your urine and blood checked every year can tell you if your kidneys are still working.

Once your kidneys fail, you may feel sick to your stomach and feel tired all the time. Your skin may turn yellow. You may feel puffy, and your hands and feet may swell from extra fluid in your body.

What happens if my kidneys fail?

First, you will need dialysis (dy-AL-ih-sis) treatment. Dialysis is a treatment that does the work your kidneys used to do. There are two types of dialysis. You and your doctor will decide what type will work best for you.

1. **Hemodialysis** (HE-mo-dy-AL-ih-sis). In hemodialysis, your blood flows through a tube from your arm to a machine that filters out the waste products and extra fluid. The clean blood flows back to your arm.

2. **Peritoneal dialysis** (PEH-rih-tuh-NEE-ul dy-AL-ih-sis). In peritoneal dialysis, your belly is filled with a special fluid. The fluid collects waste products and extra water from your blood. Then the fluid is drained from your belly and thrown away.

Second, you may be able to have a kidney transplant. This operation gives you a new kidney. The kidney can be from a close family member, friend, or someone you do not know. You may be on dialysis for a long time. Many people are waiting for new kidneys. A new kidney must be a good match for your body.

Will I know if I start to have kidney problems?

No. You will know you have kidney problems only if your doctor checks your urine for protein. Do not wait for signs of kidney damage to have your urine checked.

How can I find out if I have kidney problems?

Each year make sure your doctor checks a sample of your urine to see if your kidneys are leaking small amounts of protein called microalbumin (MY-kro-al-BYOO-min).

✎ What's It Mean?

Artery: Brings blood and waste from the bloodstream into the kidney.

Diabetic Nephropathy: The medical term for kidney problems caused by diabetes.

Dialysis: A treatment that does the work your kidneys used to do.

Glomeruli: Tiny filters throughout the kidneys.

Hemodialysis: Your blood flows through a tube from your arm to a machine that filters out the waste products and extra fluid. The clean blood flows back to your arm.

Peritoneal Dialysis: Your belly is filled with a special fluid. The fluid collects waste products and extra water from your blood. Then the fluid is drained from your belly and thrown away.

Proteinuria: When the kidneys leak protein into the urine.

The test results will tell you how well your kidneys are working.

Other tests can be done to check your kidneys. Your doctor might check your blood to measure the amounts of creatinine (kree-AT-ih-nin) and urea (yoo-REE-uh). These are waste products your body makes. If your kidneys are not cleaning them out of your blood, they can build up and make you sick.

Your doctor might also ask you to collect your urine in a large container for a whole day or just overnight. Then the urine will be checked for protein.

Chapter 32

Nerve Problems Caused By Diabetes

What can I do to prevent diabetes from damaging my nervous system?

Research has shown that people who kept their blood glucose close to normal were able to lower their risk of nerve damage.

Here is what you can do to prevent nerve damage:

- Keep your blood glucose as close to normal as you can.
- Limit the amount of alcohol you drink. [Teens should not drink any.]
- Don't smoke.
- Take care of your feet.
- Tell your doctor about any problems you have with
    - your hands, arms, feet, and legs.
    - your stomach, bowels, or bladder.
- Also tell your doctor if you
    - have problems if you have sex.

About This Chapter: Excerpted from "Prevent Diabetes Problems: Keep Your Nervous System Healthy," a publication of the National Diabetes Information Clearinghouse (NDIC), a service of the National Institute of Diabetes and Digestive and Kidney Diseases (NIDDK), National Institutes of Health (NIH), NIH Publication No. 03-4284, September 2003.

- cannot always tell when your blood glucose is too low.
- feel dizzy when you go from lying down to sitting or standing.

What can I do to take care of my feet?

- **Wash your feet in warm water every day.** Make sure the water is not too hot by testing the temperature with your elbow. Do not soak your feet. Dry your feet well, especially between your toes.

- **Look at your feet every day to check for cuts, sores, blisters, redness, calluses, or other problems.** Checking every day is even more important if you have nerve damage or poor blood flow.

- **If your skin is dry, rub lotion on your feet after you wash and dry them.** Do not put lotion between your toes.

- **File corns and calluses gently with an emery board or pumice stone.** Do this after your bath or shower.

- **Cut your toenails once a week or when needed.** Cut toenails when they are soft from washing. Cut them to the shape of the toe and not too short. File the edges with an emery board.

- **Always wear shoes or slippers to protect your feet from injuries.**

- **Always wear socks or stockings to avoid blisters.** Do not wear socks or knee-high stockings that are too tight below your knee.

- **Wear shoes that fit well.** Shop for shoes at the end of the day when your feet are bigger. Break in shoes slowly. Wear them 1 to 2 hours each day for the first 1 to 2 weeks.

- **Make sure your doctor checks your feet at each checkup.**

What does my nervous system do?

Nerves carry messages back and forth between the brain and other parts of the body. All of your nerves together make up the nervous system.

Some nerves tell the brain what is happening in the body. For example, when you step on a tack, the nerve in your foot tells the brain about the pain.

Other nerves tell the body what to do. For example, nerves from the brain tell your stomach when it is time to move food into your intestines.

How can diabetes hurt my nervous system?

Having high blood glucose for many years can damage the blood vessels that bring oxygen to some nerves. High blood glucose can also hurt the covering on the nerves. Damaged nerves may stop sending messages. Or they may send messages too slowly or at the wrong times.

Diabetic neuropathy (ne-ROP-uh-thee) is the medical term for damage to the nervous system from diabetes.

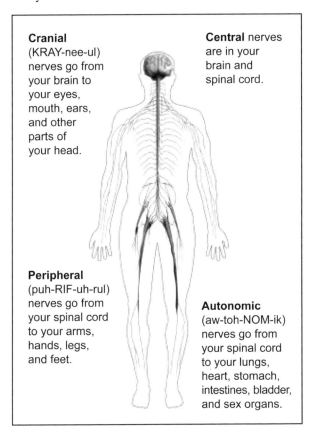

Cranial (KRAY-nee-ul) nerves go from your brain to your eyes, mouth, ears, and other parts of your head.

Central nerves are in your brain and spinal cord.

Peripheral (puh-RIF-uh-rul) nerves go from your spinal cord to your arms, hands, legs, and feet.

Autonomic (aw-toh-NOM-ik) nerves go from your spinal cord to your lungs, heart, stomach, intestines, bladder, and sex organs.

Figure 32.1. The nervous system has four main parts—central, peripheral, autonomic, and cranial. Diabetes can damage the peripheral, autonomic, and cranial nerves.

How can diabetes damage to the peripheral nerves affect me?

- **Peripheral nerves go to the arms, hands, legs, and feet.** Damage to these nerves can make your arms, hands, legs, or feet feel numb. Also, you might not be able to feel pain, heat, or cold when you should. You may feel shooting pains or burning or tingling, like "pins and needles." These feelings are often worse at night. They can make it hard to sleep. Most of the time these feelings are on both sides of your body, like in both of your feet. But they can be on just one side.

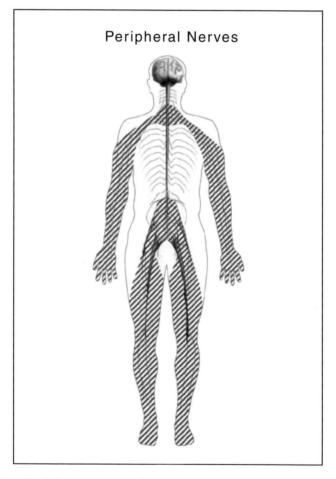

Figure 32.2. Peripheral nerves go from your spinal cord to your arms, hands, legs, and feet.

Peripheral nerve damage can change the shape of your feet. Foot muscles get weak and the tendons in the foot get shorter. You can get special shoes that are made to fit softly around your sore feet or feet that have changed shape. These special shoes help protect your feet. Medicare and other health insurance programs may pay for special shoes. Talk to your doctor about how and where to get these shoes.

How can diabetes damage to the autonomic nerves affect me?

- **Autonomic nerves help you know your blood glucose is low.** Some people take diabetes medicines that can accidentally make their blood glucose too low. Damage to the autonomic nerves can make it hard for them to feel the symptoms of hypoglycemia (hy-po-gly-SEE-mee-uh), also called low blood glucose.

  This kind of damage is more likely to happen if you have had diabetes for a long time. It can also happen if your blood glucose has been too low very often.

- **Autonomic nerves go to the stomach, intestines, and other parts of the digestive system.** Damage to these nerves can make food pass through the digestive system too slowly or too quickly. Nerve problems can cause nausea (feeling sick to your stomach), vomiting, constipation, or diarrhea.

  Nerve damage to your stomach is called gastroparesis (gas-tro-puh-REE-sis). When nerves to the stomach are damaged, the muscles of the stomach do not work well and food may stay in the stomach too long. Gastroparesis makes it hard to keep blood glucose under control.

- **Autonomic nerves go to the penis.** Damage to these nerves can prevent a man's penis from getting firm when he wants to have sex. This condition is called erectile dysfunction or impotence (IM-po-tents). Many men who have had diabetes for many years experience it.

- **Autonomic nerves go to the vagina.** Damage to these nerves prevents a woman's vagina from getting wet when she wants to have sex. A woman might also have less feeling around her vagina.

- **Autonomic nerves go to the heart.** Damage to these nerves might make your heart beat faster or at different speeds.

- **Autonomic nerves go to the bladder.** Damage to these nerves can make it hard to know when you should go to the bathroom. The damage can also make it hard to feel when your bladder is empty. Both problems can cause you to hold urine for too long, which can lead to bladder infections. Another problem can be leaking drops of urine accidentally.

- **Autonomic nerves go to the blood vessels that keep your blood pressure steady.** Damage to these nerves makes your blood move too slowly to keep your blood pressure steady when you change position. When you go from lying down to standing up or when you exercise a lot, the sudden changes in blood pressure can make you dizzy.

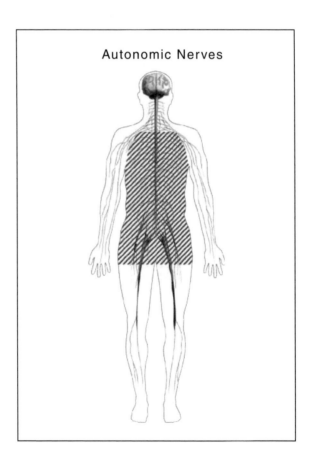

Figure 32.3. Autonomic nerves go from your spinal cord to your lungs, heart, stomach, intestines, bladder, and sex organs.

How can diabetes damage to the cranial nerves affect me?

- **Cranial nerves go to the eye muscles.** Damage to these nerves usually happens in one eye, causing double vision. This problem happens all of a sudden and usually lasts for a short time.

- **Cranial nerves go to the sides of the face.** Damage to these nerves usually happens on only one side of the face. This nerve damage causes that side of the face to hang lower or sag. Usually the lower eyelid and lips sag. This problem is called Bell's palsy. It happens all of a sudden and tends to correct itself.

How do I know if I have nerve damage?

If you have one or more of the problems mentioned in this chapter, you may have some nerve damage from diabetes. Tell your doctor about the problem. Ask your doctor what you can do to make the problem better and to stop it from getting worse.

✎ What's It Mean?

Bell's Palsy: Nerve damage in the face that causes the face (usually on only one side) to hang lower or sag. Usually the lower eyelid and lips sag.

Diabetic Neuropathy: The medical term for damage to the nervous system from diabetes.

Erectile Dysfunction (Impotence): Damage to the nerves going to the penis that can prevent it from getting firm when he wants to have sex.

Gastroparesis: Nerve damage to your stomach.

Chapter 33

Heart And Blood Vessel Problems Caused By Diabetes

What do my heart and blood vessels do?

Your heart and blood vessels make up your circulatory (SIR-kyoo-la-TOR-ee) system. Your heart is a big muscle that pumps blood through your body. Your heart pumps blood carrying oxygen to large blood vessels, called arteries (AR-ter-eez), and small blood vessels, called capillaries (KAP-ih-lair-eez). Other blood vessels, called veins, carry blood back to the heart.

What can I do to prevent heart disease and stroke?

You can do a lot to prevent heart disease and stroke.

• **Keep your blood glucose under control.** You can see if it is under control by having an A1C test at least twice a year. The A1C test tells you your average blood glucose for the past 2 to 3 months. The target for most people is below 7.

About This Chapter: Excerpted from "Prevent Diabetes Problems: Keep Your Heart and Blood Vessels Healthy," a publication of the National Diabetes Information Clearinghouse (NDIC), a service of the National Institute of Diabetes and Digestive and Kidney Diseases (NIDDK), National Institutes of Health (NIH), NIH Publication No. 03-4283, September 2003.

- **Keep your blood pressure under control.** Have it checked at every doctor visit. The target for most people is below 130/80.

- **Keep your cholesterol under control.** Have it checked at least once a year. The targets for most people are

  - LDL (bad) cholesterol: below 100

  - HDL (good) cholesterol: above 40 in men and above 50 in women

  - Triglycerides (another type of fat in the blood): below 150

> ♣ **It's A Fact!!**
> High blood glucose can cause heart and blood vessel problems.

- **Make physical activity a part of your daily routine.** Aim for at least 30 minutes of exercise most days of the week. Check with your doctor to learn what activities are best for you. Take a half-hour walk every day. Or walk for 10 minutes after each meal. Use the stairs instead of the elevator. Park at the far end of the lot.

- **Make sure that the foods you eat are "heart-healthy."** Include foods high in fiber, such as oat bran, oatmeal, whole-grain breads and cereals, fruits, and vegetables. Cut back on foods high in saturated fat or cholesterol, such as meats, butter, dairy products with fat, eggs, shortening, lard, and foods with palm oil or coconut oil.

- **Lose weight if you need to.** If you are overweight, try to exercise most days of the week. See a registered dietitian for help in planning meals and lowering the fat and calorie content of your diet to reach and maintain a healthy weight.

- **If you smoke, quit.** Your doctor can tell you about ways to help you quit smoking.

- **Ask your doctor whether you should take an aspirin every day.** Studies have shown that taking a low dose of aspirin every day can help reduce your risk of heart disease and stroke.

- **Take your medicines as directed.**

✎ Weird Words

Angina: Pain in the chest, arms, shoulders, or back, which can increase when your heart beats faster, such as when you exercise.

Arteries: Large blood vessels. The heart pumps blood to them.

Atherosclerosis: When the insides of large blood vessels become narrowed or clogged.

Capillaries: Small blood vessels. The heart pumps blood to them.

Cholesterol: A substance that is made by the body and used for many important functions. It is also found in some food derived from animals.

Heart Attack: Occurs when a blood vessel in or near the heart becomes blocked.

Peripheral Vascular Disease: When the openings in your blood vessels become narrow and not enough blood gets to your legs and feet.

Stroke: Occurs when part of your brain is not getting enough blood and stops working.

Transient Ischemic Attack (TIA): A mini-stroke.

Veins: Blood vessels that carry blood back to the heart.

How do my blood vessels get clogged?

Several things, including having diabetes, can make your blood cholesterol level too high. Cholesterol is a substance that is made by the body and used for many important functions. It is also found in some food derived from animals. When cholesterol is too high, the insides of large blood vessels become narrowed, even clogged. This problem is called atherosclerosis (ATH-uh-row-skluh-RO-sis).

Narrowed and clogged blood vessels make it harder for enough blood to get to all parts of your body. This can cause problems.

What can happen when blood vessels are clogged?

When arteries become narrowed and clogged, you may have heart problems:

- **Chest pain,** also called angina (an-JY-nuh). When you have angina, you feel pain in your chest, arms, shoulders, or back. You may feel the pain more when your heart beats faster, such as when you exercise. The pain may go away when you rest. You also may feel very weak and sweaty. If you do not get treatment, chest pain may happen more often. If diabetes has damaged the heart nerves, you may not feel the chest pain.

- **Heart attack.** A heart attack happens when a blood vessel in or near the heart becomes blocked. Not enough blood can get to that part of the heart muscle. That area of the heart muscle stops working, so the heart is weaker. During a heart attack, you may have chest pain along with nausea, indigestion, extreme weakness, and sweating.

What are the warning signs of a heart attack?

You may have one or more of the following warning signs:

- chest pain or discomfort
- pain or discomfort in your arms, back, jaw, or neck
- indigestion or stomach pain
- shortness of breath
- sweating
- nausea or vomiting
- light-headedness

Or, you may have no warning signs at all. Or they may come and go.

How does heart disease cause high blood pressure?

Narrowed blood vessels leave a smaller opening for blood to flow through. It is like turning on a garden hose and holding your thumb over the opening. The smaller opening makes the water shoot out with more pressure. In the same way, narrowed blood vessels lead to high blood pressure. Other factors, such as kidney problems and being overweight, also can lead to high blood pressure.

Many people with diabetes also have high blood pressure. If you have heart, eye, or kidney problems from diabetes, high blood pressure can make them worse.

You will see your blood pressure written with two numbers separated by a slash. For example: 120/70. Keep your first number below 130 and your second number below 80.

If you have high blood pressure, ask your doctor how to lower it. Your doctor may ask you to take blood pressure medicine every day. Some types of blood pressure medicine can also help keep your kidneys healthy.

To lower your blood pressure, your doctor may also ask you to lose weight; eat more fruits and vegetables; eat less salt and high-sodium foods such as canned soups, luncheon meats, salty snack foods, and fast foods; and drink less alcohol. [Teens should not drink any alcohol.]

What are the warning signs of a stroke?

A stroke happens when part of your brain is not getting enough blood and stops working. Depending on the part of the brain that is damaged, a stroke can cause:

- sudden weakness or numbness of your face, arm, or leg on one side of your body.

- sudden confusion, trouble talking, or trouble understanding.

- sudden dizziness, loss of balance, or trouble walking.

- sudden trouble seeing in one or both eyes or sudden double vision.

- sudden severe headache.

Sometimes, one or more of these warning signs may happen and then disappear. You might be having a "mini-stroke," also called a TIA (transient ischemic [TRAN-see-unt is-KEE-mik] attack). If you have any of these warning signs, tell your doctor right away.

How can clogged blood vessels hurt my legs and feet?

Peripheral vascular (puh-RIF-uh-rul VAS-kyoo-ler) disease can happen when the openings in your blood vessels become narrow and not enough blood gets to your legs and feet. You may feel pain in your buttocks, the back of your legs, or your thighs when you stand, walk, or exercise.

What can I do to prevent or control peripheral vascular disease?

- Don't smoke.

- Keep blood pressure under control.

- Keep blood fats close to normal.

- Exercise.

  You also may need surgery to treat this problem.

Chapter 34

Sexual And Urologic Problems Of Diabetes

Troublesome bladder symptoms and changes in sexual function are common health problems as people age. Having diabetes can mean early onset and increased severity of these problems. Sexual and urologic complications of diabetes are related to the nerve damage diabetes can cause. Men may have difficulty with erections or ejaculation. Women may have problems with sexual response and vaginal lubrication. Urinary tract infections and bladder problems occur more often in people with diabetes.

Diabetes And Sexual Problems

When you want to lift your arm or take a step, your brain sends nerve signals to the appropriate muscles. Internal organs like the heart and bladder are also controlled by nerve signals, but you do not have the same kind of conscious control over them as you do over your arms and legs. The nerves that control your internal organs are called autonomic nerves, and they signal your body to digest food and circulate blood without your having to think about it. Your body's response to sexual stimuli is also involuntary, governed by autonomic nerve signals that increase blood flow to the genitals and cause smooth muscle tissue to relax. Damage to these autonomic nerves is what can hinder normal function.

About This Chapter: Excerpted from "Sexual and Urologic Problems of Diabetes," a publication of the National Diabetes Information Clearinghouse (NDIC), a service of the National Institute of Diabetes and Digestive and Kidney Diseases (NIDDK), National Institutes of Health (NIH), NIH Publication No. 04-5135, June 2004.

Sexual Problems In Men With Diabetes

Erectile Dysfunction

Estimates of the prevalence of erectile dysfunction in men with diabetes range from 20 to 85 percent. Erectile dysfunction is a consistent inability to have an erection firm enough for sexual intercourse. The condition includes the total inability to have an erection, the inability to sustain an erection, or the occasional inability to have or sustain an erection. A recent study of a clinic population revealed that 5 percent of the men with erectile dysfunction also had undiagnosed diabetes.

Men who have diabetes are three times more likely to have erectile dysfunction as men who do not have diabetes. Among men with erectile dysfunction, those with diabetes are likely to have experienced the problem as much as 10 to 15 years earlier than men without diabetes.

In addition to diabetes, other major causes of erectile dysfunction include high blood pressure, kidney disease, alcoholism, and blood vessel disease. Erectile dysfunction may also occur because of the side effects of medications, psychological factors, smoking, and hormonal deficiencies.

If you experience erectile dysfunction, talking to your doctor about it is the first step in getting help. Your doctor may ask you about your medical history, the type and frequency of your sexual problems, your medications, your smoking and drinking habits, and other health conditions. A physical exam and laboratory tests may help pinpoint causes. Your blood glucose control and hormone levels will be checked. The doctor may also ask you whether you are depressed or have recently experienced upsetting changes in your life. In addition, you may be asked to do a test at home that checks for erections that occur while you sleep.

Treatments for erectile dysfunction caused by nerve damage, also called neuropathy, vary widely and range from oral pills, a vacuum pump, pellets placed in the urethra, and shots directly into the penis, to surgery. All these methods have strengths and drawbacks. Psychotherapy to reduce anxiety or address other issues may be necessary. Surgery to implant a device to aid in erection or to repair arteries is another option.

Retrograde Ejaculation

Retrograde ejaculation is a condition in which part or all of a man's semen goes into the bladder instead of out the penis during ejaculation. Retrograde ejaculation occurs when internal muscles, called sphincters, do not function normally. A sphincter automatically opens or closes a passage in the body. The semen mixes with urine in the bladder and leaves the body during urination, without harming the bladder. A man experiencing retrograde ejaculation may notice that little semen is discharged during ejaculation or may become aware of the condition if fertility problems arise. His urine may appear cloudy; analysis of a urine sample after ejaculation will reveal the presence of semen.

✎ What's It Mean?

Cystitis: A bladder infection.

Erectile Dysfunction: A consistent inability to have an erection firm enough for sexual intercourse.

Overactive Bladder: Bladder symptoms that may include a feeling of urinary urgency, frequency, getting up at night to urinate often, or leakage of urine (incontinence).

Neurogenic Bladder: Bladder symptoms that include difficulty urinating and complete failure to empty (retention).

Pyelonephritis: A kidney infection.

Retrograde Ejaculation: A condition in which part or all of a man's semen goes into the bladder instead of out the penis during ejaculation. This occurs when internal muscles, called sphincters, do not function normally.

Urethritis: An infection of the urethra.

Poor blood glucose control and the resulting nerve damage are associated with retrograde ejaculation. Other causes include prostate surgery or some blood pressure medicines.

Retrograde ejaculation caused by diabetes or surgery may be improved with a medication that improves the muscle tone of the bladder neck. An urologist experienced in infertility treatments may assist with techniques to promote fertility, such as collecting sperm from the urine and then using the sperm for artificial insemination.

Sexual Problems In Women With Diabetes

Decreased Vaginal Lubrication

Nerve damage to cells that line the vagina can result in dryness, which in turn may lead to discomfort during sexual intercourse. Discomfort is likely to decrease sexual response or desire.

Decreased Or Absent Sexual Response

Diabetes or other diseases, blood pressure medications, certain prescription and over-the-counter drugs, alcohol abuse, smoking, and psychological factors such as anxiety or depression can all cause sexual problems in women. Gynecologic infections or conditions relating to pregnancy or menopause can also contribute to decreased or absent sexual response.

As many as 35 percent of women with diabetes may experience decreased or absent sexual response. Decreased desire for sex, inability to become or remain aroused, lack of sensation, or inability to reach orgasm can result.

Symptoms include:

• decreased or total lack of interest in sexual relations.

• decreased or no sensation in the genital area.

• constant or occasional inability to reach orgasm.

• dryness in the vaginal area, leading to pain or discomfort during sexual relations.

If you experience sexual problems or notice a change in your sexual response, talking to your doctor about it is the first step in getting help. Your doctor will ask you about your medical history, any gynecologic conditions or infections, the type and frequency of your sexual problems, your medications, your smoking and drinking habits, and other health conditions. A physical exam and laboratory tests may also help pinpoint causes. Your blood glucose control will be discussed. The doctor may ask whether you might be pregnant or have reached menopause and whether you are depressed or have recently experienced upsetting changes in your life.

Prescription or over-the-counter vaginal lubricant creams may be useful for women experiencing dryness.

Techniques to treat decreased sexual response includes changes in position and stimulation during sexual relations. Psychological counseling, as well as Kegel exercises to strengthen the muscles that hold urine in the bladder, may be helpful. Studies of drug treatments are under way.

Diabetes And Urologic Problems

Bladder dysfunction can have a profound effect on quality of life. Diabetes can damage the nerves that control bladder function. Men and women with diabetes commonly have bladder symptoms that may include a feeling of urinary urgency, frequency, getting up at night to urinate often, or leakage of urine (incontinence). These symptoms have been called overactive bladder. Less common but more severe bladder symptoms include difficulty urinating and complete failure to empty (retention). These symptoms are called a neurogenic bladder. Some evidence indicates that this problem occurs in both men and women with diabetes at earlier ages than in those without diabetes.

Neurogenic Bladder

In neurogenic bladder, damage to the nerves that go to your bladder can cause it to release urine when you do not intend to urinate, resulting in leakage. Or damage to nerves may prevent your bladder from releasing urine properly and it may be forced back into the kidneys, causing kidney damage or urinary tract infections.

Neurogenic bladder can be caused by diabetes or other diseases, accidents that damage the nerves, or infections.

Symptoms of neurogenic bladder include:

• urinary tract infections.

• loss of the urge to urinate when the bladder is full.

• leakage of urine.

- inability to empty the bladder.

Your doctor will check both your nervous system (your brain and the nerves of the bladder) and the bladder itself. Tests may include x-rays and an evaluation of bladder function (urodynamics).

Treatment for neurogenic bladder depends on the specific problem and its cause. If the main problem is retention of urine in the bladder, treatment may involve medication to promote better bladder emptying and behavior changes to promote more efficient urination, called timed urination. Occasionally, people may need to periodically insert a thin tube called a catheter through the urethra into the bladder to drain the urine. Learning how to tell when the bladder is full and how to massage the lower abdomen to fully empty the bladder can help as well. If urinary leakage is the main problem, medications or surgery can help.

Urinary Tract Infections

Infections can occur in any part of the urinary tract. They are caused when bacteria, usually from the digestive system, reach the urinary tract. If bacteria are growing in the urethra, the infection is called urethritis. The bacteria may travel up the urinary tract and cause a bladder infection, called cystitis. An untreated infection may go farther into the body and cause pyelonephritis, a kidney infection. Some people have chronic or recurrent urinary tract infections.

Symptoms of urinary tract infections may include:

- a frequent urge to urinate.
- pain or burning in the bladder or urethra during urination.
- cloudy or reddish urine.
- fatigue or shakiness.
- in women, pressure above the pubic bone.
- in men, a feeling of fullness in the rectum.

If the infection is in your kidneys, you may be nauseous, feel pain in your back or side, and have a fever. Since frequent urination can be a sign of high blood glucose, you and your doctor should also evaluate recent blood glucose monitoring results.

Your doctor will ask for a urine sample, which will be analyzed for bacteria and pus. If you have frequent urinary tract infections, your doctor may order further tests. An ultrasound exam provides images from the echo patterns of sound waves bounced back from internal organs. An intravenous pyelogram (IVP) uses a special dye to enhance x-ray images of your urinary tract. Another test, called cystoscopy, allows the doctor to view the inside of the bladder.

♣ **It's A Fact!!**
You can lower your risk of sexual and urologic problems by keeping your blood glucose, blood pressure, and cholesterol close to the target numbers your doctor recommends.

Early diagnosis and treatment are important to prevent more serious infections. To clear up a urinary tract infection, the doctor will probably prescribe an antibiotic based on the bacteria in your urine. Current recommendations are for a full 7-day course of antibiotic treatment in people with diabetes, instead of the shorter course used for other people. Kidney infections are more serious and may require several weeks of antibiotic treatment. Drinking plenty of fluids will help prevent another infection.

Will I Experience Sexual And Urologic Problems Sooner Or Later?

Risk factors are conditions that increase your chances of getting a particular disease. The more risk factors you have, the greater your chances of developing that disease or condition. Diabetic neuropathy, including related sexual and urologic problems, appears to be more common in people who:

- have poor blood glucose control.

- have high levels of blood cholesterol.

- have high blood pressure.

- are overweight.

- are over the age of 40.

- smoke.

What Can I Do To Prevent Diabetes-Related Sexual And Urologic Problems?

Being physically active and maintaining a healthy weight can also help prevent the long-term complications of diabetes. Smoking is a particular problem, and quitting will improve your health in many ways. For example, if you quit smoking, you can lower your risk not only for nerve damage but also for heart attack, stroke, and kidney disease.

Chapter 35

Diabetes And Eating Disorders

Because both diabetes and eating disorders involve attention to body issues, weight management, and control of food, some people develop a pattern in which they use the disease to justify or camouflage the disorder. Because the complications of diabetes and eating disorders can be serious, even fatal, responsible, healthy behavior is essential.

How many people have both an eating disorder and diabetes?

We are not sure, but the combination is common. Some clinicians think that eating disorders are more common among folks with diabetes than they are in the general population. Research is currently underway to find out if this is so.

Does diabetes cause anorexia nervosa or bulimia?

No, diabetes does not cause eating disorders, but it can set the stage, physically and emotionally, for their development. Once people develop eating disorders, they can hide them in the overall diabetic constellation. This makes treatment and even diagnosis difficult. In some of these cases the eating disorder has gone undetected for years, sometimes coming to light only when life-altering complications appear.

About This Chapter: "Diabetes and Eating Disorders" reprinted with permission of ANRED: Anorexia Nervosa and Related Eating Disorders, Inc., http://www.anred.com, April 2005.

What are some of those life-altering complications?

Blindness, kidney disease, impaired circulation, nerve death, and amputation of limbs. Death, of course, is the ultimate life-altering complication.

People who have both diabetes and an eating disorder eat in ways that would make their doctors wince. Many believe that being fat, a perceived immediate threat, is far worse than the consequences noted above which may never happen, or if they do, will happen years down the road. Like Scarlett O'Hara, they will worry tomorrow.

Many of these people superstitiously believe they will escape complications. They are wrong.

What is the main mechanism that connects diabetes and eating disorders?

People who take insulin to control their diabetes can misuse it to lose weight. If they cut back the required dosage, blood sugar will rise and spill over into the urine. These folks will lose weight, but the biochemical process is particularly dangerous. Reducing insulin causes body tissues to dissolve and be flushed out in urination.

Once diabetics discover that they can manipulate their weight this way, they are reluctant to stop even if they know about potential consequences because weight loss is rewarding in our fat-phobic culture. They decide to maintain the weight loss, and that decision can serve as the trigger for a full-blown eating disorder.

What are the similarities between diabetes and eating disorders?

Both demand that people pay close attention to body states, weight management, types and amounts of food consumed, and the timing and content of meals. Both encourage people to embrace some foods as "safe" and "good" and fear others as "dangerous" and "bad."

Control is a central issue in both diabetes and eating disorders. Diabetics may feel guilty, anxious, or out of control if their blood sugar swings more than a few points. Anorexics and bulimics may feel the same way if their

✦ It's A Fact!!
People with eating disorders are pre-occupied with weight, food, and diet. So are folks with diabetes.

weight fluctuates. People with both problems may become consumed with strategies to rigidly control both weight and blood sugar.

Children with diabetes may have parents they perceive as overprotec-tive and overcontrolling. The parents of young people with eating disorders are often described in similar terms. In both kinds of families over involve-ment and enmeshment can lead children to rebellion and dramatic, poten-tially catastrophic, acts of independence.

People with eating disorders are preoccupied with weight, food, and diet. So are folks with diabetes. In fact, the latter can use their diabetes to hide anorexia or bulimia because, after all, they are supposed to be watching what they eat, and they can blame poorly controlled diabetes for alarming weight loss.

Are there any other problems related to a combination of diabetes and eating disorders?

Yes. When people misuse insulin to lose weight, sometimes that weight loss seems to improve diabetes, at least temporarily, by reducing or eliminat-ing the need for insulin. It's interesting to note that starvation was a primary treatment for diabetes before commercial production of supplemental insu-lin. This weight loss method is not without problems, however. If continued, the person experiences life-threatening organ failure and death.

What kind of treatment should people who have both diabetes and EDs have?

Getting them into treatment is the first step. Many of these folks are embarrassed to admit that they have been doing something as unhealthy as an eating disorder. Often they defiantly hang onto starving and stuffing be-haviors in spite of real threats to life and health. Families sometimes collude by denying that anything is wrong.

Nevertheless, it is important to begin treatment early. Eating disorders can be treated, and people do recover from them, but the longer symptoms are ignored, the harder it is to turn them around and the harsher the effects on the body.

The best treatment is team treatment. That means that many professionals are involved with the patient and perhaps with the family as well: a physician to manage the diabetes and the effects of starving and stuffing, a mental health therapist to help define and deal with underlying emotional issues, a family therapist to help the family, and a dietitian to provide nutritional counseling and education.

The first priority is restoration of physical health. For people with anorexia that means weight gain back to healthy levels. For both anorexics and bulimics the next step is implementation of balanced, varied, and healthy meal plans that provide adequate calories and nutrients. After physical health is stabilized, treatment can focus on the underlying psychological issues.

Most treatment for eating disorders is outpatient, but if the patient is suicidal, severely depressed, or in any kind of medical danger, hospitalization is appropriate until the crisis has passed. Medication may be used to ease depression and anxiety, but it must be carefully monitored by a physician.

In Summary

Diabetes and eating disorders are a nasty combination with very real potential for catastrophic complications, including death. The good news, however, is that in most cases diabetes can be controlled, and eating disorders can be treated. Many people recover from anorexia nervosa and bulimia, but almost always professional help is required.

If you are concerned about yourself, arrange right now to talk to your physician. Don't let shame or embarrassment stop you from telling the truth. The doctor has heard your story many times before. Ask for a referral to a mental health professional who works with people with eating disorders. Contact that person and ask for an evaluation. Then follow up on any treatment recommendations that come from the evaluation. Other people have made this journey successfully. You can too.

Chapter 36

Diabetes And Alcohol Use

Underage kids shouldn't drink alcohol. It's illegal.

But the danger alcohol poses to kids with diabetes goes beyond the sad and familiar toll it takes among American teens, in terms of car crashes and alcohol poisonings. It poses a double threat to teens with diabetes, because it can also cause life-threatening blood glucose lows. So let's get right to the facts.

According to American Diabetes Association's clinical guidelines, men should have no more than two alcoholic drinks each day, and women should have no more than one. It's important to know that one drink is the equivalent of one beer, a five-ounce glass of wine, or one and one-half-ounces of gin, vodka, rum, or whiskey. Drinking more than double this amount can be what's called "binge drinking," which is consuming a large amount of alcohol over a short period of time, even if it's done only a few days a month. When your liver is called upon to clear this large volume of alcohol from your blood, it is unable to produce the sugar or glucose that it delivers into your bloodstream, especially overnight when you are not eating. This is where the danger for people with diabetes begins.

About This Chapter: "Underage Drinking," by Judi Zielke. Copyright © 2004 American Diabetes Association. From *Diabetes Forecast*, September 2004. Reprinted with permission from The American Diabetes Association.

The glucose-lowering effect of alcohol can last anywhere from 8 to 12 hours after you consume it. Typically, these are the hours you would be sleeping after an evening event. If your blood glucose level drops dangerously low while you sleep and you are sedated from the alcohol, you may not awaken to treat your low blood glucose. If alcohol is consumed with little or no food, low blood glucose (hypoglycemia) can develop at very mild intoxication levels.

If you start to experience low blood glucose levels when you are still with others, they may confuse your symptoms with intoxication. You may even confuse the effects of the alcohol with feelings caused by a drop in your blood glucose levels. This could result in a potentially serious situation, such as becoming unconscious and needing an ambulance ride to the emergency room.

To prevent problems that can result from mixing alcohol and diabetes, here are some guidelines:

Never drink on an empty stomach. Alcohol is safest when taken with food. Have your scheduled meal before the party, and snack on carbohydrate-containing foods such as crackers or pretzels.

Pour your own drink if possible so that you can control the amount of alcohol you consume. Avoid sweet liqueurs such as kahlua, because of the high sugar content. Use mixes such as club soda, tomato juice, or diet sodas instead of juices or regular soda. Drink slowly.

Stick with drinks with lower alcohol content such as light beers.

Be prepared for low blood glucose. Carry a quick-acting carbohydrate such as glucose tablets, Lifesavers, or hard candy.

Let a friend you'll be with know that you have diabetes, and what symptoms to watch for when your blood glucose is dropping. This person must understand that you'll need something containing carbohydrates even if you only appear mildly intoxicated. He or she must also know that if you appear ill, or are vomiting, you'll need professional medical attention. The risk of a hypoglycemic coma from alcohol is very real.

Monitor your blood glucose every few hours when you are drinking alcohol, especially if you are being physically active, perhaps when dancing or playing ball at the beach.

Before you get into bed, set your alarm to ring midway through the night. When it rings, check your blood glucose. If it's below 100, eat a carbohydrate snack.

Have a snack before you go to bed, even if your blood glucose level is high at that time. Remember that your liver will be clearing the alcohol from your body and not releasing any glucose for hours after you've stopped drinking.

Drinking alcohol is a privilege of adulthood. The guidelines listed above hold for anyone with diabetes who drinks alcohol. Your safety is the main concern when drinking, because the alcohol may cloud your judgment. And always remember to have a designated driver—alcohol and driving do not mix.

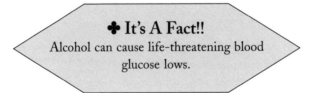

♣ It's A Fact!!
Alcohol can cause life-threatening blood glucose lows.

Chapter 37

Diabetes And Tobacco Use

While quitting smoking or chewing tobacco may not be easy, it could be the best thing you can do to prevent the complications of diabetes.

Your Blood Sugar Level

Tobacco raises your blood sugar level. This makes it harder to control your diabetes. Nicotine and other products in tobacco smoke make it more difficult for insulin to work properly. Additionally, chewing tobacco is high in sugar.

Your Eyes

If you use tobacco, it is likely you will experience even more trouble with your sight. Diabetes can block the tiny blood vessels in the eyes. This condition is called retinopathy. Tobacco makes your eyes even less healthy.

Your Teeth

If you smoke or chew tobacco and have diabetes, you will have a greater chance of developing gum disease and losing your teeth. The sugar and harsh chemicals in tobacco eat away at the teeth and gums.

About This Chapter: Information in this chapter is from "Tobacco and Diabetes." Reprinted with permission from the Utah Department of Health Tobacco Prevention and Control Program, http://www.tobaccofreeutah.org. © 2004 Utah Department of Health. All rights reserved.

Your Nerves

If you have diabetes, smoking will increase the risk of nerve damage in all parts of your body, causing numbness and sometimes pain. This may occur because tobacco damages the blood vessels that carry oxygen and nutrients to the nerves. Smoking slows down blood flow and blocks blood vessels in the penis, and nerve damage reduces sensation. If you are a man who uses tobacco and has diabetes, you are more likely to experience problems having an erection.

Your Heart

You are more likely to have a heart attack or stroke and three times more likely to die of heart disease if you have diabetes and use tobacco. The nicotine in all tobacco products increases your heart rate. The carbon monoxide in tobacco smoke reduces oxygen in the blood. Tobacco causes blood vessels to constrict. This means your heart has to work harder to pump blood throughout the body. Smoking makes blood cells stick together and chemicals in tobacco harm blood vessels so that fat attaches to the vessel walls even faster, causing them to clog. Uncontrolled blood glucose levels also cause blood vessels to narrow. Together, these symptoms lead to heart attack and stroke.

Your Kidneys

Even in people without diabetes, smoking triples the chances of developing kidney disease. Smoking increases blood pressure and affects chemicals in the body that control kidney function. Medications that successfully prevent kidney failure in most nonsmoking diabetics (ACE Inhibitors) may not help tobacco users with diabetes.

Your Feet

It is extremely unusual for a person with diabetes to have a leg amputated due to blocked blood vessels unless they use tobacco. Tobacco slows the circulation in the smaller blood vessels. People with diabetes are already more likely to suffer from poor circulation in their feet and legs. Tobacco use can also aggravate foot ulcers, foot infections, and blood vessel disease in the legs.

✔ **Quick Tip**
How To Quit

- Set a quit date. Within 2 weeks is best.

- Tell family and friends you are quitting. Social support helps!

- Think about what you can learn from past quit attempt experiences. What worked? What didn't?

- Anticipate challenges. Symptoms such as irritability, cravings, insomnia, and coughing may occur for 2 to 3 weeks after quitting.

- Remove tobacco products. In addition, ask family members who use tobacco not to smoke around you or leave their tobacco products where you can get them during your quit attempt.

- Ask your doctor about medications to help you quit. Using Zyban (bupropion SR) or nicotine replacement therapy (NRT) will double or triple your chance of quitting successfully by reducing nicotine withdrawal symptoms, including cravings.

- Enroll in a support program to help you quit.

Don't be too tough on yourself if quitting takes a few tries. The average smoker or chewer must make several quit attempts before they quit for good. Each attempt increases the odds that the next try will be successful. Learn from unsuccessful quit attempts. What were the most common triggers that caused you to slip?

- Persons

- Places

- Things

- Situations

For each trigger list two new ways you can deal with the trigger so you won't slip. Repeat the process if the new ways don't work.

Is It True That I Will Gain Weight If I Quit Using Tobacco?

Some people—but not all—do gain weight as they quit. However, this weight gain is usually limited to between 5 and 10 pounds, and some of this weight gain can be prevented.

Nicotine increases metabolism in a way that is harmful to health. It causes body tension, accelerates the heart rate, increases blood pressure, and causes physical agitation. When you quit smoking, your metabolism returns to normal rates and your body returns to the weight that it would have been had you never smoked. Weight gain is usually limited to 10 pounds or less and can be delayed by using bupropion SR or NRT.

You might gain 3 to 5 pounds due to water retention during the first week after quitting, but it will go away after a week.

Tobacco use reduces the ability to smell, so food is naturally more appealing when you quit. Since food tastes better, some quitters tend to eat more than they did as tobacco users. Is this preventable? Yes!

Tobacco users develop a habit of frequently putting their hands to their mouth to smoke or chew. When they give up tobacco, some people continue this habit, substituting food for tobacco. Is this preventable? Yes!

Cravings for cigarettes or chew during nicotine withdrawal can be confused for hunger pangs. Is this preventable? Yes!

Healthy Ways To Minimize Weight Gain

- **Become more physically active.** In addition to helping control weight, exercise may help relieve the stress and depression caused by purging nicotine from the body. Some studies have shown that increased physical activity actually improves quit rates in addition to reducing weight gain.

- **Gradually improve eating habits.** Strict dieting does not prevent weight gain in quitters and makes it harder to quit using tobacco.

- **Replace smoking with healthy activities.** Snack on fruit or sugarless gum to satisfy any sweet cravings. Replace the action of holding cigarettes with activities like doodling, working puzzles, knitting, twirl-ing a straw, or holding a pen or pencil. Relieve tension by meditating, taking a walk, soaking in the tub, or taking deep breaths.

- **Drink plenty of fluids, especially water and juice.** Drinking lots of water both cleanses the body of nicotine, decreasing the duration and severity of withdrawal symptoms, and helps people feel more full so they don't overeat. But avoid caffeinated beverages, which may make nicotine withdrawal worse.

- **Try not to panic about modest weight gain.** Some weight gain is the healthy result of returning to normal metabolism. The health risks of smoking are far greater than the risks of gaining 5 to 10 pounds. You would have to gain about 100 pounds after quitting to make your health risks as high as when you smoked.

Part Four

Day-To-Day Living With Diabetes

Chapter 38

Eating And Diabetes

Why do you need to eat healthy foods?

- For energy to learn, play, and live

- To grow at a healthy rate

- To help keep your blood sugar or glucose (GLOO-kos) levels in balance—not too high or too low

- To help you lose weight slowly if you need to

- To keep your body working properly

- To help you avoid other health problems caused by diabetes

Do kids with diabetes need special foods?

No, they don't. Meals that are healthy for kids with diabetes are great for everyone in the family.

How does food affect your body?

Food is the fuel that our bodies use for energy. The three main sources of fuel are carbohydrates (CAR-boh-HY-drate), protein, and fat. The body

About This Chapter: Excerpted from "Eat Healthy Foods," National Diabetes Education Program (NDEP), National Institutes of Health (NIH), NIH Publication No. 03-5295, August 2005.

changes them into glucose for energy or stores them as fat. A car uses gas for energy—we use glucose. Eating a balance of foods that contain carbohydrate (carbs), protein, and fat every day will help your blood glucose stay in balance and keep your weight where you want it to be.

Carbs are a good source of energy for our bodies. Many foods contain carbs. Some are better for you than others. If you eat too many carbs at one time, your blood glucose may go up too high. Learn to eat the right amount at meal and snack times to keep your blood glucose in balance.

✔ Quick Tip

To create a healthy meal plan you should do the following:

- Eat a variety of foods to get a balanced intake of the nutrients your body needs—carbohydrates, proteins, fats, vitamins, and minerals.

- Make changes gradually because it takes time to accomplish lasting goals.

- Reduce the amount of fat you eat by choosing fewer high-fat foods and cooking with less fat.

- Eat more fiber by eating at least 5 servings of fruits and vegetables every day.

- Eat fewer foods that are high in sugar like fruit juices, fruit-flavored drinks, sodas, and tea or coffee sweetened with sugar.

- Use less salt in cooking and at the table. Eat fewer foods that are high in salt, like canned and packaged soups, pickles, and processed meats.

- Eat smaller portions and never skip meals.

- Learn about the right serving sizes for you.

- Learn how to read food labels.

Source: Excerpted from "Recipe and Meal Planner Guide," National Diabetes Education Program (NDEP), National Institutes of Health (NIH), cited September 2005; available online at www.ndep.nih.gov/diabetes/MealPlanner/en_intro.htm.

These are good carb choices. They have lots of fiber.

- Whole grain foods
- Fresh fruits and vegetables from every color of the rainbow—red, orange, yellow, white, green, blue, and purple

Choose these carbs less often:

- White bread
- White rice
- Sweetened fruit drinks
- Sweets and desserts

Protein foods help to build strong muscles and bones. Protein foods do not make the blood glucose go up like some carbs do. Having protein in your meal can help you feel less hungry.

Foods that are a good source of protein include:

- Meat and poultry without the extra fat or skin
- Fish, low-fat cheese, and eggs
- Dried peas or beans such as kidney, white, split, or blackeye
- Soy products and nuts

Fats are a good source of fuel for the body and help you grow. Fat does not make blood glucose go up, but too much fat can make you gain weight.

Choose fats that keep your heart healthy:

- Small portions of salad dressing, low-fat mayonnaise, and margarine in a plastic tub
- Nuts, olives, and vegetable oil
- Avocados

Choose these high fat foods less often. They are not healthy for your heart:

- Butter, stick margarine, and regular mayonnaise
- Fried foods such as potato chips and french fries

- Meats with fat on them, including bacon and lunch meats

- Cakes, cookies, pies, and other desserts

What about sugar, sweets, and desserts?

Everyone likes the taste of sweet foods. Small amounts of foods that contain sugar can be part of a healthy meal plan. Sugary foods include soda pop, sweetened fruit drinks, syrup, honey, and candy.

Desserts such as cakes, muffins, pies, cookies, and ice cream contain a lot of fat as well as sugar. If you choose to eat any of these sweet foods, just have a small amount at the end of a healthy meal. Have a piece of fruit if you are still hungry.

Drink water, sugar-free soda pop, and sugar-free fruit drinks if you are thirsty—instead of regular soda pop, sweetened fruit drinks, and sports drinks that are all high in sugars.

How much should you eat?

Your height, weight, age, whether you are a boy or a girl, and how active you are will affect how much food you need to eat each day to stay at a healthy weight. Everyone is different. Talk to your doctor or dietitian about how much to eat, especially if you need to lose weight.

It's best to spread your food out over the day and eat breakfast, lunch, and dinner and a couple of snacks as well. You will have a ready supply of energy and you won't get too hungry.

If you take in more food than your body burns, you will gain weight. If you take in less food than your body burns, you will lose weight. Being active and eating smaller amounts of food and fewer sweet or fatty foods can help overweight kids lose weight in a healthy way. You will keep your heart healthy, too.

Putting It All Together

- Eat meals and snacks at about the same time each day. Try not to skip meals.

- Be physically active for at least 60 minutes almost every day.

- Drink more water instead of juice or soda.

- Learn more about foods and how much you need to eat.

- Ask your doctor or dietitian for help.

- Take the right amount of insulin or pills at the right times if you need them to help manage your diabetes.

☞ Remember!!

It's not always easy to eat healthy foods when others seem to eat whatever they want. Follow the tips in this chapter and know that it will make a difference in your life.

Chapter 39

Eating Out When You Have Diabetes

Whether it's the local pizza joint after a game, the food court at the mall, or barbecued ribs on your best friend's back porch, eating out is probably a part of your social scene.

You don't want to miss out on these activities just because you have to watch what you eat, and the good news is you don't have to. You can pretty much eat the same foods as your friends and family—you just have to keep track of what you eat and eat certain foods in moderation.

Which restaurant should I choose?

If you're choosing where to eat, think about the places that offer you the most options—even fast-food places have healthy choices on their menus.

Don't worry—you're not limited to places that serve only soy burgers and carrot sticks. If you can order a meal that includes a good balance of proteins, fats, and carbohydrates, you're doing OK. But if you find that certain restaurants don't offer many vegetable choices or that they only serve fried food that's covered in cheese, you might want to pick a place that offers more options.

About This Chapter: Information in this chapter is from "Eating Out When You Have Diabetes." This information was provided by TeensHealth, one of the largest resources online for medically reviewed health information written for parents, kids, and teens. For more articles like this one, visit www.TeensHealth.org, or www.KidsHealth.org. © 2005 The Nemours Center for Children's Health Media, a division of The Nemours Foundation.

You might find that there are more healthy breakfast choices—like yogurt, fresh fruit, and scrambled eggs—for you at the diner than at the coffeehouse, so convincing your friends to chow down on diner food is one option. But if your friends prefer the coffeehouse, one alternative is to buy something to drink and bring a snack in your backpack or purse that's easy to eat discreetly, like pretzels or raisins. Some people may be embarrassed or worried that the manager might give them a hard time, though. If you think you may get caught in a situation like this, you can talk about what to do with your doctor or dietitian and how to adjust your meal plan or insulin doses.

What should I order?

When it's time to order, follow the same rules for food content and portion sizes that you follow at home. Your meal plan probably calls for you to eat a good balance of proteins, fats, and carbs. Usually, you can get all of the nutrients you need at a restaurant, too. These tips can help:

> **✔ Quick Tip**
> Whenever possible, look for nutritional facts on the meal you plan to order—like calorie, carbohydrate, and fat content. This information is available in many chain restaurants (you may need to ask for it) or online. Or ask your server what's in the food you're eating.

- **Change and rearrange.** To get a well-balanced meal in a restaurant, feel free to substitute certain ingredients or side orders (for example, you could substitute salad for fries). Don't feel weird about it—people ask for substitutions all the time. You can also ask for a different preparation, like having your chicken broiled instead of fried.

- **Watch the sides.** Avoid foods with sauces or gravy, and ask for low-fat salad dressings on the side.

- **Pick your own portion.** Restaurant portions often offer enough food to feed your entire crew, but try to eat the same portion of food that you'd eat at home. Either eat only part of your order and take the rest home or split it with a friend.

- **Master menu lingo.** Watch out for words like "jumbo," "supersize," "deluxe," or "value" when eating at your favorite fast-food joint or the food court at the mall. Instead, order junior- or regular-sized sandwiches and sides.

- **Split with a friend.** Are you hungry for some fries? Order a healthy sandwich and side salad for yourself and sneak a few of your friend's fries instead of ordering your own. And dividing an entrée or sandwich between friends also helps keep portion sizes under control.

- **Go light on buns and crusts.** Choose thin-crust pizza over the deep-dish pie and skip double burgers and extra-long hot dogs to keep carb intake under control. And keep in mind that English muffins, bread, and small buns often contain fewer calories and fat than croissants and biscuits.

The same tips apply to eating at your school cafeteria. To be a healthy eater at school, make sure you pick a variety of healthy foods and stop to think about when you're getting full.

What should I bring with me?

When you go out to eat, you should bring the things you take with you everywhere, like testing supplies, snacks, and medications. A quick-reference guide to food content and portions can make choosing healthy foods a little easier. (If you don't have one, you can get one from your doctor or dietitian.) If you use things like artificial sweeteners or fat-free spreads, bring them along, too.

If you take insulin, eating later than usual might mean making a few adjustments to your medicine schedule. There's no need to stay home, though—if you'll be eating later than usual, hold off on your insulin injection, eat a small snack at your normal mealtime, and take the insulin later.

Do you have questions about how to make eating out even easier? Talk to your doctor or dietitian.

Chapter 40

Stay At A Healthy Weight To Improve Blood Sugar Levels And Prevent Diabetes Complications

Why is staying at a healthy weight good for kids?

A healthy weight means you are not too fat or too thin. Your doctor may have said that you should not gain more weight or that you need to lose a few pounds. If you have diabetes and are overweight, you are not alone.

The steps you take to manage your weight will help you feel better and may improve your blood sugar or glucose (GLOO-kos) levels. Staying at a healthy weight when you are young can help you manage your weight for life. It also can help prevent problems like heart disease and high blood pressure.

How can you get to a healthy weight?

If your doctor says you need to lose some weight, you need to eat fewer calories each day and be more active. Here are some ways to succeed.

- **Be active almost every day** for 60 minutes to burn up extra calories and get fit. Play tag or go for a bike ride instead of playing computer games. Ask a friend or family member to join you on a walk instead of watching TV.

About This Chapter: Excerpted from "Stay at a Healthy Weight," National Diabetes Education Program (NDEP), National Institutes of Health (NIH), NIH Publication No. 03-5295, August 2005.

- **Cut some calories.** The number of calories in a food shows how much energy you can get from it. To lose weight, you need to eat about 200 to 300 calories less than usual each day. Here are some simple ways to cut calories:
    - Drink water instead of a big glass of sweetened fruit drink or regular soda pop. You can cut about 150 calories.
    - Eat a small serving of french fries instead of a big one and cut about 250 calories.
    - Eat a piece of fruit instead of a candy bar. You will cut about 200 calories.
- **Eat smaller portions** of food and drink water at meals and snack time.
- **Drink lots of water.** It has no calories. Sugar-free fruit drinks or sugar-free soda pop are also good choices when you are thirsty.
- **Ask your doctor to help you find a dietitian** or a diabetes educator. He or she can help you and your family make the best food choices.

If you eat less and get more active, you should lose about one pound a month and feel great. It's best to be slow and steady in your weight loss because you are still growing. Ask your doctor to help you.

Very low-calorie diets are not healthy for growing children and teens. Kids who do not eat enough food may not grow or develop the right way.

What about breakfast?

One bowl of whole grain cereal, nonfat or low-fat milk, and a piece of fruit are a great way to start the day. You can do better at school when you eat breakfast.

When you don't have much time before school, try a couple of slices of whole grain toast with a tablespoon of peanut butter, or a hard-boiled egg, or a piece of low-fat cheese.

A small breakfast bar and a glass of nonfat or low-fat milk is another fast meal that can go a long way.

What about school lunches?

If you get your lunch at school, choose fried foods less often. Choose nonfat or low-fat milk instead of chocolate milk and a piece of fresh fruit instead of a cookie.

Many schools have salad bars. Choose high fiber vegetables and fruits and low-fat protein foods. Use a small amount of low-calorie dressing.

Small deli or sub sandwiches made with lean turkey or beef are healthy choices, too. Use mustard or a little low-fat mayonnaise.

If you have time in the morning, you could pack a lunch of healthy foods to take to school. Or you could make your lunch the night before.

What about after school snacks?

Most kids need an after school snack. Choose healthy snacks. The trick is not eating too much. Use a small plate or a bowl for your snack instead of eating out of the bag or box. It will be easier to keep track of how much you eat. It's best not to snack while watching TV or at the computer—you may eat too much.

✔ Quick Tip
Healthy Eating Tips You Can Try

- Take your time when you eat. Wait 10 to 15 minutes before eating second helpings at mealtime. It takes about 15 minutes for your stomach to tell your head that you are full.

- Ask if you can help plan, shop, or make the family meals sometimes. This can be fun for the whole family.

- Fill up half of your plate with salad or vegetables. Use small amounts of butter, margarine, or salad dressing.

- If you eat sugary foods, sweets, desserts, or candy, eat only a small serving at the end of a meal. Don't eat them very often.

Snack ideas:

- A piece of fresh fruit

- Half a turkey or ham sandwich, easy on the mayo

- A small bowl of whole-grain cereal with nonfat or low-fat milk

- A small bowl of vegetable soup and a few crackers

- One small tortilla with one or two slices of shredded low-fat cheese or turkey

- 3 to 6 cups of low-fat microwave popcorn, one handful of pretzels, or a few rice cakes

Remember to drink a couple of glasses of water, too.

What about fast-food restaurants?

Try not to super-size your meals, unless you plan to share them with your family or a friend. Order smaller child-sized meals and drink water, nonfat or low-fat milk, or diet soda pop.

A grilled chicken sandwich or a simple hamburger is a better choice than a burger that is covered with secret sauce, cheese, and bacon. A baked potato with a little butter or sour cream is a good choice, too.

If you are eating pizza, order thin or medium crust instead of deep dish or stuffed crust pizzas. Eat only one or two slices and add a salad with a little dressing.

Try a small bag or a handful of baked chips or pretzels instead of the regular kind of chips.

☞ **Remember!!**
The key to success is to have the whole family make healthy food choices and to be as active as you can.

Chapter 41

Physical Activity And Diabetes

Why is being active so important?

Exercise is good for everyone, whether you have diabetes or not. Being active keeps your body healthy and strong. It can help you stay at a weight that's right for you or help you lose weight slowly.

Physical activity can make you feel better if you're in a bad mood, relax you, and help you sleep well. If you have diabetes, exercise can help your body use glucose (GLOO-kos) for energy and lower your blood sugar (glucose).

What types of activity are good to do?

There are many ways you can stay active.

- Walk the dog, take a hike, or ride a bike.

- Roller skate, in-line skate, or ice skate.

- Dance, swim, or jog.

- Check out an aerobics tape from the library and work out at home.

- You can play basketball, baseball, softball, golf, soccer, tennis, or volley-ball.

About This Chapter: Excerpted from "Be Active," National Diabetes Education Program (NDEP), National Institutes of Health (NIH), NIH Publication No. 03-5295, August 2005.

- Take the stairs instead of the elevator, skip rope, fly a kite, throw a disc, or play hopscotch.

Think of other things you can do and just move it! Don't forget to have fun!

Make exercise a part of your daily life. Be active with a friend or family member—it is easier and more fun when you have a buddy.

What should you do before exercising?

Talk to your doctor about what physical activity is good for you.

- Ask if you need to check your blood glucose before starting any activity or after you are done.

✔ Quick Tip
Make a list of some things you like to do. Hang it in your room as a reminder.

- Ask if the medicine you take can make your blood glucose get too low during exercise. If so, keep a snack with you when you exercise.

How much exercise do you need to do?

If you haven't been very active, start slowly. Try a few minutes each day. Slowly work up to 60 minutes almost every day. Pick an activity you like to do.

How can your family and friends help?

Ask your family members and friends to be active with you—it's good for everyone and helps to get rid of stress. It's a great way for families to spend time together, too. Ask your family to take a walk after dinner, instead of watching TV. Instead of playing computer games, put on some music that everyone can dance to. Help your mom or dad carry groceries, clean the house, cut the grass, do garden work, rake leaves, or shovel snow.

☞ Remember!!

If you have diabetes, you need to choose healthy foods, be active every day, take your medicine, check your blood glucose as often as your doctor suggests, and stay at a healthy weight. Taking care of your diabetes will help you stay healthy, feel better, and keep your blood glucose where you want it to be.

What if you don't like to exercise?

There are a lot of things you can do to be more active. Try these: do sit-ups, lift light weights, or jump rope while you watch TV. Take the stairs when you can, run around during recess at school, or walk fast around the mall a few times when you go shopping. You don't have to play a sport or go to a gym.

Don't get upset if you can't do a lot or if you get out of breath at first— keep trying. Any amount of activity will help and you can add a little more each week.

Chapter 42

Athletes And Diabetes

In Brief: Athletes with diabetes require intensive diabetes management to balance insulin, carbohydrate intake, and the effects of exercise. Effective care of active patients who have diabetes starts with a targeted preparticipation exam. Decreasing the insulin dosage may be necessary for heavier exercise programs if carbohydrate supplementation alone is insufficient. The documented risk for either hypoglycemia or ketoacidosis requires careful planning for training or competition. Analysis of high-risk activities is essential to determine which may need to be modified, diminished, or restricted.

Approximately 16 million people with diabetes mellitus live in the United States. Of the 10% who have type 1 diabetes (also known as insulin-dependent or juvenile-onset diabetes), about half are under 20 years old, with the prevalence in this age group estimated at 260 per 100,000. The other 90% have type 2 diabetes, also called non-insulin-dependent or adult-onset diabetes. Wider recognition of the benefits of intensive diabetes management is a recent phenomenon, but there has long been a philosophy among diabetes specialists to advise patients to become more physically active in hopes of improving their diabetes control and enhancing their quality of life. The

About This Chapter: Reprinted with permission from Draznin, Martin, "Type 1 Diabetes and Sports Participation," *The Physician and Sportsmedicine*, December 2000, 28 (12): p.49 (8). Copyright © 2000 the McGraw-Hill Companies. Reviewed October 2005 by David A. Cooke, M.D., Diplomate, American Board of Internal Medicine.

development of type 2 diabetes can be significantly delayed by exercise and by maintaining an active lifestyle. We should anticipate increasing numbers of athletes with diabetes to be involved at all levels of participation and competition because the incidence of both types of diabetes is increasing. This chapter, however, focuses on active people who have type 1 diabetes.

The Effects Of Physical Activity On Metabolism

During physical activity, exercising muscles significantly increase their use of oxygen and of substrates such as muscle and liver glycogen, muscle triglycerides, and free fatty acids. These substrates are mobilized by the action of epinephrine, glucagon, cortisol, and growth hormone. In a healthy person, blood glucose concentration continues to be regulated by these hormones and by insulin so that it remains within an appropriate range.

The brain requires a minimum concentration of plasma glucose for maintaining normal functions, including surveillance of the space surrounding the athlete, judgment, and consciousness. Because of this requirement, hypoglycemia is severely maladaptive during exercise. At the other extreme, the kidneys may not be able to maintain adequate circulating plasma volume if hyperglycemia and glycosuria diminish the ability to deliver oxygen to exercising muscles. Additionally, the metabolism of fatty acids for energy results in the generation of ketones that, in excessive concentrations, depress plasma pH and interfere with the normal function of nerves and muscles, including the heart. In short, in the healthy person, the concerted action of several hormones allows for as much as a 20-fold increase in oxygen consumption without departure of several key substances from a narrow range of plasma concentrations needed for normal function.

Type 1 diabetes may involve normal hormonal responses mediating the release of fuels or degrees of deficiency of glucagon and/or epinephrine response. The availability of insulin to counter excess elevation of plasma glucose is not under the exquisite control seen in a healthy individual. To increase glucose absorption and insulin levels in a diabetic person, capillary blood flow increases in exercising muscle to enhance the accessibility of insulin receptors to the insulin in circulation. Also, blood flow to the insulin injection sites increases. With the loss of the tight normal control of circulating insulin and glucose, dangerously disabling hypoglycemia may occur during exercise. Another risk is delayed hypoglycemia occurring several hours after exercise, possibly during sleep.

Conversely, if preexisting mild ketosis or significant hyperglycemia is present at the start of vigorous physical activity, ketoacidosis may be precipitated. This occurs when the so-called counter-insulin hormones raise the level of glucose and free fatty acids more rapidly than the enhanced insulin uptake by muscle receptors, and the exercise-induced increase of insulin concentration can act to suppress lipolysis and ketogenesis. By careful assessment of metabolic control, athletes with type 1 diabetes must learn to regulate the injection of correctly adjusted doses of insulin and ingest appropriate nutrients to duplicate the system that runs automatically and without conscious effort in healthy athletes.

Exercise Benefits In Diabetes

There are obvious social benefits to exercise and sports participation: peer relationships developed and enhanced by shared experiences, enhanced self-esteem and confidence from mastery of a skill, learning about teamwork, character, and courage, etc. In addition, some studies suggest health benefits for athletes with type 1 diabetes. Aerobic circuit training helped adolescents improve cardiorespiratory endurance, muscle strength, lipid profiles, and glucose regulation. Research showed that adults with type 1 diabetes safely reduced cardiovascular risk factors such as abdominal fat content, blood pressure, and adverse lipid levels by exercising 135 min/wk. Researchers were enthusiastic about the benefits of resistance training for individuals with diabetes but cautioned that when there is microvascular disease, such as retinopathy, athletes should avoid lifting excessively heavy weights, which could increase intravascular pressure. Maintaining good metabolic control is also important. Other studies, however, suggest that the changes in type 1 diabetes are not that substantial or lasting.

Finally, several athletes have told their stories of self-improvement, advocacy, how they learned to deal with insulin balances, and a bit of the frustration felt as they discovered how to manage their diabetes and their sports participation by trial and error. Because each patient's body chemistry

✎ What's It Mean?

Autonomic Neuropathy: A type of neuropathy affecting the lungs, heart, stomach, intestines, bladder, or genitals.

Basal Rate: A steady trickle of low levels of longer-acting insulin, such as that used in insulin pumps.

Gastroparesis: A form of neuropathy that affects the stomach. Digestion of food may be incomplete or delayed, resulting in nausea, vomiting, or bloating, making blood glucose control difficult.

Glucagon: A hormone produced by the alpha cells in the pancreas. It raises blood glucose. An injectable form of glucagon, available by prescription, may be used to treat severe hypoglycemia.

Glycogen: The form of glucose found in the liver and muscles.

Glycosuria: The presence of glucose in the urine.

Hyperglycemia: Excessive blood glucose. Fasting hyperglycemia is blood glucose above a desirable level after a person has fasted for at least 8 hours. Postprandial hyperglycemia is blood glucose above a desirable level 1 to 2 hours after a person has eaten.

Hypertension: A condition present when blood flows through the blood vessels with a force greater than normal. Also called high blood pressure. Hypertension can strain the heart, damage blood vessels, and increase the risk of heart attack, stroke, kidney problems, and death.

Hypoglycemia: A condition that occurs when one's blood glucose is lower than normal, usually less than 70 mg/dL. Signs include hunger, nervousness, shakiness, perspiration, dizziness or light-headedness, sleepiness, and confusion. If left untreated, hypoglycemia may lead to unconsciousness. Hypoglycemia is treated by consuming a carbohydrate-rich food such as a glucose tablet or juice. It may also be treated with an injection of glucagon if the person is unconscious or unable to swallow. Also called an insulin reaction.

Diabetic Ketoacidosis: An emergency condition in which extremely high blood glucose levels, along with a severe lack of insulin, result in the breakdown of body fat for energy and an accumulation of ketones in the blood and urine. Signs of DKA are nausea and vomiting, stomach pain, fruity breath odor, and rapid breathing. Untreated DKA can lead to coma and death.

Ketone: A chemical produced when there is a shortage of insulin in the blood and the body breaks down body fat for energy. High levels of ketones can lead to diabetic ketoacidosis and coma. Sometimes referred to as ketone bodies.

Ketosis: A ketone buildup in the body that may lead to diabetic ketoacidosis. Signs of ketosis are nausea, vomiting, and stomach pain.

Neuropathy: Disease of the nervous system.

Nephropathy: Disease of the kidneys. Hyperglycemia and hypertension can damage the kidneys' glomeruli. When the kidneys are damaged, protein leaks out of the kidneys into the urine. Damaged kidneys can no longer remove waste and extra fluids from the bloodstream.

Peripheral Neuropathy: Nerve damage that affects the feet, legs, or hands. Peripheral neuropathy causes pain, numbness, or a tingling feeling.

Diabetic Retinopathy: Diabetic eye disease; damage to the small blood vessels in the retina. Loss of vision may result.

Subcutaneous: Putting a fluid into the tissue under the skin with a needle and syringe.

Triglyceride: The storage form of fat in the body. High triglyceride levels may occur when diabetes is out of control.

Vitreous: The clear gel that lies behind the eye's lens and in front of the retina.

Source: "Diabetes Dictionary," National Diabetes Information Clearinghouse (NDIC), a publication of the National Institute of Diabetes and Digestive and Kidney Diseases (NIDDK), National Institutes of Health (NIH), NIH Publication No. 04-3016, November 2003; available at http://diabetes.niddk .nih.gov/dm/pubs/dictionary.

and circumstances are unique, it is difficult to make generalizations about what kind of insulin regimen is needed for a particular sport. Most of the day-to-day care and assessment of diabetes is done by the athletes and their families; therefore, their physicians provide more counseling and education than direct care.

Preparticipation Assessment

The basics of preparticipation assessment of the athlete with diabetes are identical to those of any other athlete. All aspects of general health and fitness (cardiovascular health, flexibility, freedom from injury, neurologic integrity, absence of any critical paired organ, etc.) should be assessed for suitability for that particular sport for that participant (Table 42.1).

Table 42.1. The Preparticipation Exam, History, and Evaluation for Patients Who Have Type 1 Diabetes

General Exam and Sports History

Is overall health adequate?

Cardiovascular and pulmonary assessment

Musculoskeletal assessment

Neurologic assessment

Any current illness issues that preclude participation?

Any specific concerns such as old injuries or illness that make participation risky?

Any loss of one of paired organs?

Assess Level of Diabetes Self-Care Skills and Knowledge

Review of glycated hemoglobin levels and blood glucose logs (careful record keeping is required for successful adaptation of care to be feasible)

Any episodes of hypoglycemia or ketoacidosis? Were they adequately resolved?

Knowledge of treatment for hypoglycemia and sick day regimen

Understanding of the actions of each component of the insulin regimen and peak times

Accuracy of techniques of injection, monitoring of blood glucose, pump use, etc.

Understanding of carbohydrate counting:

Complications of diabetes that would preclude certain sports activities should then be determined. Retinopathy would make it risky to engage in activities that rapidly or explosively elevate intraocular pressure that may cause hemorrhage into the vitreous humor. Bleeding from damaged retinal capillaries during Valsalva's maneuver while lifting heavy weights or from collisions with other athletes also poses a risk. An examination for early signs of retinopathy should be done by an expert at least once a year.

Peripheral neuropathy increases the risk of injuries because of lack of sensation or abnormalities of gait. Autonomic neuropathy heightens the risk for lack of cardiac responsiveness to rapidly changing needs for increased cardiac output and may interfere with the absorption of nutrients. Gastroparesis could also make absorption of carbohydrates unpredictable.

Table 42.1. Continued.

    Extra carbohydrate needed for exercise (calculate g/hr)

    How to decrease insulin for exercise

How Will the Sports Activity Affect the Diabetes?

Is there a preseason camp? If so, what is the duration of training and time during the day?

What is the duration and timing of training during the season?

Do coaches, athletic trainers, and others have adequate knowledge of the diabetic athlete's needs?

Is support of the athlete's needs by the coaches, athletic trainers, and team appropriate?

Are adequate resources available to meet the needs of the athlete?

How often and how far does the team travel?

    How is diabetes care altered by travel? Will there be overnight trips?

    How will travel times affect regular meal times and what food will be available?

    How will diabetic emergencies be handled aboard a bus, plane, train, or van?

What sort of changes occur during competition?

    What needs to be done to prepare and arrange for them?

The presence of nephropathy and hypertension could also be risky. It is not known how many individuals with diabetic neuropathy or nephropathy are currently attempting to pursue sports; thus, the nature and magnitude of the risks to those individuals is unclear.

Next, a careful history should be taken of how the athlete manages diabetes so that adjustments can be made to match the changes caused by training and participation in the sport in question. It is also important to learn whether previous sports-related difficulties (injury, poor performance, etc.) were due to problems with managing diabetes and whether the athlete understands the mechanism of the problem. Important characteristics of the athlete such as emotional stability, maturity, dedication to training, and acceptance of the need to master care of diabetes should also be evaluated. It is vital as well to ensure the adequacy of support systems such as family, coaches, and athletic trainers, all of whom may need to be involved in any problems that need resolution to allow the athlete to participate at an optimal level and with reasonable safety.

High-Risk Sports

Any sport involves a risk of injury. This risk is likely to be magnified by inattention or loss of coordination, such as during an episode of hypoglycemia. In extremely risky sports and activities, the risks are much higher. For example, rock and mountain climbing may expose participants to a lethal danger of falling if their concentration lapses, so a climber with diabetes would have to ensure that hypoglycemia was not going to happen. Skydiving requires continuous focus of attention as well.

Scuba diving is another potentially high-risk activity; thus, its suitability for individuals with diabetes has been studied. For example, military diving is not allowed in Great Britain for people with type 1 diabetes, and in the United States they cannot join the military at all. Sport scuba diving may be safe with adequate preparation and a skilled partner who can handle trouble with diabetes during the dive. A carefully designed plan to prevent and remedy any hypoglycemia without undue risk to the diving partner should be in effect before diving is attempted. Any sport that tends to expose the athlete to significant periods of isolation from outside sources of assistance—for example, a long-range dogsled race—would have to be similarly assessed.

Sports in which the danger of inattention or loss of motor control would endanger others, in addition to endangering the athlete with diabetes, should not be entered into casually; in fact, many would oppose any participation in such activities by athletes with diabetes. Proper sports etiquette suggests soliciting in advance of participation the assent and support of anyone who may be affected by an adverse event.

Preparation For Sports

A thorough understanding of the nature of the training, practices, and competition, and in the potential effects on metabolic control in diabetes, is necessary to craft a plan for safe and productive training and optimal performance. Some factors to consider are:

- how many hours and what kind of activity will be endured;

- what times of day and on how many days per week it will be done;

- how the exercise timing matches insulin peaks;

- whether there are provisions for administering extra carbohydrate to treat hypoglycemia if the sources of carbohydrate planned and taken by the athlete before and during practice or competition are insufficient;

- who has the responsibility for assisting the athlete with severe hypoglycemia and whether that person has the resources needed, such as a glucagon emergency kit, and appropriate training;

- whether the coaches and athletic trainers are willing to accommodate the athlete's occasional needs to do things differently from the other athletes;

- whether the coaches and trainers support the athlete's efforts to participate.

Given a thorough preparticipation evaluation, it is possible to tailor diabetes care to allow for very active sports participation, including extremely difficult participation, such as an Ironman triathlon. Intensive diabetes management with multiple daily injections of insulin, or an insulin pump, and numerous checks of blood glucose throughout the day will give a clearer picture of the effects of exercise (Table 42.2).

Table 42.2. Matching Insulin Treatment Schedules With Exercise
Schedules

Treatment Type	Advantages	Disadvantages
Standard— 2 shots: mixed intermediate and short insulins	Easy to perform	Poor match with exercise, rigid time restraints, least likely to give good metabolic control and health
Intensive— 3 or more shots a day	Better control, more flexible timing, less hypoglycemia in the evening	More frequent testing, harder to learn
Extended— insulin zinc suspension or glargine for basal plus lispro for meals with either	Least amount of time rigidity, most protection against hypoglycemia, excellent metabolic control	Much more effort to master and do well
Continuous infusion (pump)	Most flexible (no injections most days), low hypoglycemia risk overnight, best metabolic control	Needs expensive device,* harder to master, must remove pump for some activities

*Pumps cost $4,000 to $6,000. Infusion sets are $4 to $6 each and can be
used up to 2 days.

A standard strategy for moderate training schedules is to offset the increased efficiency of insulin use by ingesting 15 g of carbohydrate for every half hour of moderate aerobic exercise. Monitoring of blood glucose during practices of several hours' duration is advised. Adjusting insulin downward may be necessary for heavier exercise programs if carbohydrate supplementation alone is insufficient, or if the extra food intake is too uncomfortable and limiting to the athlete. It may be necessary, in some cases, to decrease the total insulin dosage by a third or more during sports seasons, unless the athlete is active at the same level all year. In that case, the dosage may not need to be modified. Blood glucose should be checked more often early in the training season to assess how to balance insulin, carbohydrate intake, and exercise. (See section titled "Success Stories of Insulin Adjustments.")

It is critical to counsel the athlete to check for and prevent delayed hypoglycemia that often occurs after muscle and liver glycogen has been depleted and not replenished during exercise. Another way to lessen the risk of this problem is to avoid the use of intermediate-acting insulin during the afternoon or early-evening hours by shifting its injection to bedtime, or by replacing intermediate-acting insulin with a long-acting insulin option that does not "peak."

Newer insulins include a synthetic aspart that, like lispro, is very rapidly utilized and gone from the circulation and glargine, an extended insulin zinc suspension that is advertised to be administered once daily. Ultralente works more safely if given twice a day. Glargine has not had the exposure yet to determine whether it truly is a once-a-day basal insulin.

Testing is done before meals and at bedtime regardless of the type of insulin used. To establish the dose (given by injection or by pump) for long-acting insulin plus lispro for meals, the patient also tests blood glucose 2 hours after each meal for 3 to 4 weeks. Careful record keeping will determine if assumptions are correct and which doses work best.

Proper use of an insulin pump, with its adjustable basal rates for differing sensitivities to insulin, should offer even more protection against nocturnal hypoglycemia. Pumps are about the size of pagers and are worn on the belt of regular clothing or in a sports pack. In the past, pump use in sports was very complicated, but some current models can be worn even while swimming if placed in a waterproof pack. The infusion set is a soft plastic catheter that remains in the skin for up to 2 days attached to the pump by a flexible plastic tube.

For collision sports and those in which the athlete experiences extreme degrees of flexing, twisting, and contact near the area of skin where the infusion set is attached, it may be necessary to inject subcutaneous insulin and detach the pump during the activity. The infusion set remains in place. The amount of insulin injected should initially be the same number of units the pump would have delivered over the time it is to be replaced. Adjustments to the dosage are then made until the blood glucose level remains in a suitable range.

♣ It's A Fact!!
Success Stories Of Insulin Adjustments

I had the pleasure of watching televised portions of the Hawaii Ironman Triathlon in 1984 during which Brad Carlson, an athlete who has type 1 diabetes, participated with the support of his physicians. He removed his insulin pump and took subcutaneous insulin before the swimming portion of the race, then put the pump back into service for the bicycle ride and the run. He was required to make numerous stops to check his blood glucose level and to discuss with his physicians what to do next. His comment on finishing the race was that he would log a better time if he didn't have to check in as much. He subsequently did exactly what he predicted—the next time he competed, he did his own adjustments and improved his performance.

A 14-year-old skater switched her insulin from her usual mixture (intermediate- and short-acting insulin at breakfast, short-acting at the evening meal, and intermediate-acting at bedtime) to a twice-a-day extended insulin zinc suspension for basal insulin and lispro, a very short-acting insulin, for meal coverage. She needed to awaken and eat at 4 a.m. to get on the ice to practice before school. Additionally, the high school had a 10:30 a.m. lunchtime that gave other students with diabetes some difficulty. She found it fit her schedule perfectly.

A 16-year-old swimmer in had numerous instances of hypoglycemia. He is a very hard-working athlete and would push himself beyond the safe limits of his insulin shots. He often needed to stop in the middle of practice to eat, and felt very weak and panicky when hypoglycemia occurred in the middle of the pool. Fortunately, he never lost consciousness. He switched to using an insulin pump that he could detach from the infusion set during practice and competition. He has not had trouble with hypoglycemia caused by over-rapid absorption of insulin since he switched to the pump method and is now much safer in the water.

An elite high school tennis player was happy with an extended insulin zinc suspension injection twice a day and regular insulin for meal coverage but switched his short insulin to lispro. This suited him even better since the wait between injection and eating is only 10 minutes with lispro rather than the 40 minutes for the regular insulin. He then noticed that he had more bedtime hyperglycemia when using lispro for dinner coverage. He independently adjusted his regimen to include half lispro and half regular insulin with dinner, and his hyperglycemia resolved without hypoglycemia.

In addition to preventing hypoglycemia during and after exercise, it is also necessary for the athlete with diabetes to monitor blood glucose prior to exercising to avoid precipitating hyperglycemia and ketoacidosis. These may occur if exercise is done in the absence of adequate insulin.

Signs of hypoglycemia include apparent loss of concentration and focus, shaking or shivering, and loss of consciousness. A designated person must be available at all practices and competitions to look for signs of hypoglycemia, check athletes for hypoglycemia in case there is any question of it, and help manage hypoglycemia when athletes are unable to treat themselves. This person should know how to administer rapidly absorbed forms of glucose to conscious athletes and glucagon when athletes are unable to safely swallow glucose. In cases of hypoglycemia with carbohydrate depletion, glucagon is less effective. Plans for intravenous fluids containing glucose may be needed as well. Many hospitals have diabetes educators who provide training classes, and family members involved in day-to-day care are also knowledgeable.

Some manufacturers claim that glucose gels can be absorbed in adequate quantity by just rubbing them on the gums, but the volume needed to provide adequate glucose is on the order of several milliliters, so swallowing is required. Thus, to protect the airway from aspiration of the gels, the athlete who is being treated with gels should be responsive and cooperative.

The Physician As Educator

Participation in sports often enhances the health and quality of life for those with diabetes. Knowledge of the specific metabolic changes that exercise induces, and how to adjust the management of insulin and nutrition, will allow these benefits to be safely enjoyed by diabetic athletes. The goals of the physician caring for an individual with diabetes should include allowing participation in as wide a range of life-enhancing activities as can be safely done. Because the care of diabetes is done mostly by the patient and family, the physician's key role in facilitating sports activities is as an educator.

Chapter 43

Diabetes And Sports Nutrition

Type 1 diabetes is a condition in which the body is unable to produce insulin. Without insulin, the body's ability to use glucose as a fuel source is impaired. Does this mean that people with Type 1 diabetes have to give up dreams of a successful sports career? With good management, it is possible to participate in sporting activities, even at an elite level, with this condition.

How Does Type 1 Diabetes Affect Metabolism?

Insulin is a hormone produced in the pancreas. It has a number of important functions in the body, including a regulatory effect on carbohydrate metabolism. Insulin stimulates glucose to be taken up by body cells and used for fuel. It inhibits the release of glucose from glycogen in the liver and stimulates the synthesis of muscle glycogen after exercise. In the absence of diabetes, insulin is released according to the body's needs and the concentration of glucose in the blood is kept within a small range. People with Type 1 diabetes do not produce insulin. The body is therefore unable to use glucose properly as a fuel source and starts to rely on fat and protein as fuel. This causes blood glucose levels to rise excessively and toxic byproducts from fat breakdown (ketones) to build up in the blood. If untreated, this can be fatal.

About This Chapter: Information in this chapter is from "Type 1 Diabetes and Sports Nutrition," 2004. Reproduced with permission from the Australian Sports Commission. Reviewed October 2005 by David A. Cooke, M.D., Diplomate, American Board of Internal Medicine.

How Is Type 1 Diabetes Treated?

Type 1 diabetes requires regular insulin injections. The amount and timing of insulin administration needs to be matched to factors such as food intake, individual metabolism, and activity level. Blood glucose levels must be monitored regularly to ensure an appropriate amount of insulin is given. Poor use of insulin will result in abnormal blood glucose levels.

Hypoglycemia—Low Blood Glucose

Occurs when too much insulin is present causing too much glucose to be taken up by the body's cells and too little glucose to be released from the liver. Symptoms include sweating, rapid heart rate, drowsiness, shaking, confusion, poor coordination, and nausea. If untreated, hypoglycemic coma occurs. This is a potentially fatal condition that requires rapid medical assistance.

✎ What's It Mean?

Glucose: One of the simplest forms of sugar.

Glycogen: The form of glucose found in the liver and muscles.

Ketone: A chemical produced when there is a shortage of insulin in the blood and the body breaks down body fat for energy. High levels of ketones can lead to diabetic ketoacidosis and coma. Sometimes referred to as ketone bodies.

Pancreas: An organ that makes insulin and enzymes for digestion. The pancreas is located behind the lower part of the stomach and is about the size of a hand.

Source: "Diabetes Dictionary," National Diabetes Information Clearinghouse (NDIC), a publication of the National Institute of Diabetes and Digestive and Kidney Diseases (NIDDK), National Institutes of Health (NIH), NIH Publication No. 04-3016, November 2003; available at http://diabetes.niddk.nih.gov/dm/pubs/dictionary.

Hyperglycemia—High Blood Glucose

Occurs when too little insulin is present. Too much glucose is released from the liver and cells cannot take up glucose adequately. Symptoms include restlessness, poor concentration, fatigue, thirst, muscle cramps, drowsiness, and nausea. In the long term, regular hyperglycemia increases the risk of complications related to diabetes including cardiovascular, kidney, and eye problems.

How Does Exercise Affect Diabetes Management?

Factors such as muscle contraction, increased blood flow, and increased body temperature cause the body to be more responsive or sensitive to insulin during exercise. Therefore, in people who do not have diabetes, insulin levels decrease during exercise. People with Type 1 diabetes usually need to adjust their insulin dose to account for a reduced requirement for insulin during exercise. Management of diabetes varies for each individual. Regular monitoring of blood glucose levels and trial and error (under the supervision of your diabetes specialist) is needed to understand and manage each individual's response to exercise. However, in general, the following factors need to be considered:

- **Intensity and duration of exercise.** Pre-exercise insulin dose generally needs to be reduced when exercise extends beyond 30 minutes. The level of reduction varies for each individual, but in general, the longer the period of exercise, the greater the reduction required. Adjustments to insulin should be made with the guidance of your diabetes specialist, especially in the early stages of management.

- **Degree of metabolic control before exercise.** It is easier to manage and predict the body's response to exercise when metabolic control is good. It is dangerous to commence exercise when blood glucose levels are high and ketones are present in the urine.

- **Type and dose of insulin injected before exercise.** It is common practice to use a mixture of short- and long-lasting insulin to manage diabetes. It is necessary to predict the peak period of insulin activity to avoid excessive levels of insulin injection during exercise.

- **Site of insulin injection.** Insulin absorption is increased in exercising muscles. The abdomen is usually the preferred site for insulin injection prior to exercise.

- **Timing of previous meal.** The amount and type of food consumed influence insulin requirements.

How Does Type 1 Diabetes Affect Dietary Requirements?

In general, people with Type 1 diabetes have the same dietary requirements as the general population—a varied diet with plenty of fruit, vegetables, legumes, bread and cereals, moderate amounts of fish, meat, poultry, eggs and dairy products, and smaller amounts of foods high in fat, refined sugar, and alcohol.

Including foods with a low glycemic index (GI) is thought to assist with blood glucose control. Glycemic index is a tool used to rank foods according to their immediate effect on blood glucose levels. Carbohydrate-containing foods that are broken down quickly, releasing glucose rapidly into the blood stream, are known as high GI foods. Conversely, carbohydrate-containing foods that break down slowly, releasing glucose gradually into the blood stream, are known as low GI foods. People with diabetes (and the general population) are encouraged to consume a variety of low GI foods each day. Examples of low GI foods include the following:

- fresh fruit—apples, bananas, pears, mangos and grapes
- multigrain bread
- pasta
- milk
- low fat fruit yogurt
- baked beans

✔ Quick Tip
People with Type 1 diabetes are encouraged to adjust their insulin regime according to food intake and activity levels rather than distorting their food intake to suit the insulin dose.

For further information on GI, speak to your diabetes specialist.

Blood glucose control is usually better when a consistent eating pattern is adopted with regular meals and snacks.

How Does Type 1 Diabetes Affect Sport Nutrition Strategies?

General sports nutrition strategies are similar whether or not you have diabetes. Managing Type 1 diabetes and competing successfully requires a commitment to trying different food and fluid combinations in and around exercise. It is impossible to provide a single set of guidelines that will suit all people with Type 1 diabetes. This chapter outlines some issues to consider. You will need to work with your diabetes specialist and use trial and error to find the best approach for you.

> ### ♣ It's A Fact!!
> Blood glucose levels should be monitored closely before exercise. It may be necessary to consume extra carbohydrate before commencing exercise if blood glucose levels are low.

Eating Before Training And Competition

As for all athletes, a carbohydrate-based pre-exercise meal 1–3 hours before exercise is recommended. This may need to be followed up with a small snack closer to exercise. Theoretically, it may help to include a low GI food in the pre-exercise meal. However, research on non-diabetic athletes has not been able to indicate a clear benefit of having a low GI pre-exercise meal, provided sufficient total carbohydrate is consumed, and research on diabetic athletes has not been conducted.

It is important for people with Type 1 diabetes to ensure blood glucose levels are at an appropriate level before commencing exercise—ideally between 4–8 mmol/L (72–144 mg/dL). Exercising with high blood glucose levels disrupts normal metabolic control and will elevate levels even further. Apart from being dangerous, this will result in poor performance. In general, exercise should be postponed if blood glucose levels are above 10–14 mmol/L (180–252 mg/dL), especially if ketones are present in the urine.

Blood glucose control is easier if you have a consistent training routine. It becomes more difficult in competition situations when the start time is unknown or the length of the event varies. Being attuned to the symptoms of hypo- and hyperglycemia and regular monitoring is necessary in these situations.

Eating During Training And Competition

Eating during exercise depends on the duration and intensity of exercise. In general, additional carbohydrate should be considered as exercise approaches one hour or more. Research suggests 30–60 g of carbohydrate per hour will aid performance. Usually it is not necessary to have extra insulin if you eat during exercise. Choices such as sports drinks that provide fluid and carbohydrate are a convenient option for most exercise situations. Other options such as carbohydrate gels, fruit and sports bars may also be tolerated. If additional carbohydrate is required during exercise, it is better to consume small amounts frequently rather than leave it until the last minute.

Eating After Training And Competition

General sports nutrition recovery strategies are the same as for non-diabetic athletes. Fuel and fluid used during exercise needs to be replaced. The increased insulin sensitivity caused by exercise lasts for several hours after exercise. Therefore the risk of hypoglycemia persists for some time. Delayed hypoglycemia can occur 4–48 hours after exercise. Preventing delayed hypoglycemia involves making sure you consume sufficient carbohydrate before, during, and after exercise. It may also be necessary to reduce the next insulin dose after exercise. It is helpful to monitor your blood glucose levels frequently after exercise. Inconveniently, delayed hypoglycemia often occurs during the night. If this occurs regularly, it can exacerbate fatigue in athletes. Waking up feeling very tired and groggy in the morning may indicate you have experienced a "hypo" during the night. This is a sign that you need to increase blood glucose monitoring after similar exercise sessions in the future.

Alcohol inhibits the release of glucose from the liver, therefore increases the risk of hypoglycemia. Consuming alcohol also impairs the ability to recognize the symptoms of hypoglycemia.

Little research is available directly on athletes with diabetes. However, it is possible that people with Type 1 diabetes have a reduced ability to store glycogen after exercise. This may be an issue when strenuous training sessions are held within a short period of time (less than 24 hours apart).

✔ Quick Tip

Try any new strategies during training sessions when it is easier to monitor the effects on blood glucose control.

Is Carbohydrate Loading Safe For People With Diabetes?

Carbohydrate loading is dependent on insulin availability, and therefore, requires good diabetic control. It is necessary to adjust insulin administration to account for the increased carbohydrate intake and the effects of an exercise taper. Regular blood glucose monitoring is essential when carbohydrate loading. Carbohydrate loading should not be attempted if blood glucose control is poor. Seek advice from your diabetes specialist and sports dietitian if you wish to use this method.

Controlling Blood Glucose Levels During Competition

Excitement and nerves surrounding competition are almost inevitable. A side effect of excitement is the release of hormones such as adrenalin and cortisol. These hormones stimulate the release of glucose from the liver and reduce the effectiveness of insulin. This can cause fluctuating blood glucose levels. Ways to avoid or cope with this include the following suggestions:

- Emulate your race/competition preparation in training (including physical preparation and recovery, and nutrition strategies).

- Try and practice some relaxation techniques (correct breathing techniques, muscle relaxation techniques, music, or talk to a sports psychologist).

- Write your routine down on paper before the event so you don't forget your routine amongst all the excitement.

You may need to consider taking slightly more insulin for competition day or using a more intensive insulin routine (that is, frequent and small doses of short acting insulin). This should be practiced and planned in conjunction with your diabetes specialist.

Carbohydrate intake on competition day should not be sacrificed to try and reduce blood glucose levels. The result could be insufficient energy for competition—there is no benefit to doing this. Forward planning and practice will help avoid this situation.

Blood Glucose Levels And Strength Training

Strength-oriented exercise (for example, lifting weights or even sports like tae kwon do) generally requires short, repetitive, and intensive bursts of movement. This type of exercise can provoke a hormone response known as the "fight or flight" or "adrenalin" response that can temporarily raise blood glucose levels. Currently, it is not known whether this temporary hyperglycemia from weight training has any long-term effect and management of this response is difficult and still controversial.

Decreasing carbohydrate intake in an attempt to avoid the anticipated hyperglycemia might jeopardize performance during exercise and increase the risk of delayed hypoglycemia after exercise. Increasing your insulin dose after exercise to reduce blood glucose levels may increase the risk of delayed hypoglycemia once the adrenalin response has worn off.

Regular blood glucose monitoring is important so that you are aware of how your body responds to strength exercise. You should consult your diabetes specialist if you are concerned about your blood glucose response to weight training and seek guidance on the best way for you to respond.

Supplements And Type 1 Diabetes

Before considering use of any dietary supplement, you are strongly advised to see your diabetes specialist or sports dietitian. Even supplements entrenched in sports such as sports drinks can be misused and contribute to poor sports performance. Learning how to use dietary supplements properly is a skill, and seeking advice from a sports dietitian can help you to get it right. Most sports supplements are poorly researched and little, if any, research is conducted on athletes with diabetes. It is important to discuss the potential effects of any product with a knowledgeable person before using any supplement.

Weight Loss And Body Fat Loss With Type 1 Diabetes

Achieving a weight goal, reducing body fat, or just maintaining weight, should be a planned and realistic process in order to avoid the temptation for fad diets or radical weight loss or gain. This is very important in diabetes as rapid weight loss can lead to severe hypoglycemia, fatigue, and poor exercise performance. These negative consequences of rapid weight loss defeat the purpose of reducing weight or body fat in the first place.

As a person with Type 1 diabetes, it is important to consider the impact of what you eat in relation to your blood glucose levels as a priority rather than how it immediately affects your weight. Rapid fluctuations in weight affect your health much more significantly than someone without diabetes.

A sports dietitian can help you to plan your nutrition requirements if weight loss is an issue for your sport.

Travel

Athletes with diabetes need to pack ample supplies of insulin and testing equipment. Supplies need to be packaged in a container that protects from heat stress and physical damage. Consider packing half your supplies in your hand luggage and the rest in your checked in luggage.

> ☞ **Remember!!**
> It is important to train with a partner who is aware of the problems and knows how to treat hypoglycemia. Coaches of athletes with diabetes need to understand the effects of diabetes on athletic performance and be familiar with their athlete's management plans. They should also be prepared to treat hypoglycemia.

Responsible Management

Maintaining good diabetic control will maximize the benefits from training. It is important to persevere to understand your own metabolic response and develop a management strategy. Regular consultation with your diabetes specialist is important. Athletes with diabetes need to plan for the management of hypoglycemia.

Thinking About Starting A Sport?

If you are contemplating getting into a sport, then you should first seek a medical assessment (complications screening) by your diabetes specialist. A sports physician can also offer an assessment based on the requirements of your chosen sport/s and help guide the pace at which you get into your sport.

Want To Improve Your Performance In Your Current Sport?

There are many factors related to diabetes that can influence physical performance as well as all the factors unrelated to diabetes that influence performance. You may need to adopt a team approach so you manage your diabetes and your exercise performance simultaneously. Be sure to involve your diabetes specialist, sports physician, and coach to help maximize your sports performance and manage your diabetes.

Monitoring Diet And Training

A training diary is probably the most important and useful tool you can embrace as an athlete. Consider combining your diabetes-monitoring tool with your training diary in order to monitor both diabetes and non-related diabetes factors simultaneously. There are a number of commercial sports training diary programs available through the Internet. Alternatively, you could create your own in a spreadsheet using the suggested headings below. Your diabetes specialist can assist you to properly record diabetes-related responses to exercise.

Date

It's always handy to know when the event took place.

Training Times

Exercising at different times during the day may affect your body's response during or after exercise.

Nature Of The Exercise

Recording the type, duration and intensity of exercise enables you to more accurately reflect on the nature of the exercise you undertook. Keeping a record will help you or your dietitian/diabetes specialist/coach to work out whether your nutritional strategies are appropriate. It will also enable you to see whether your training is adequate or excessive over time.

Blood Glucose Levels

Regular blood glucose testing is recommended as part of your usual diabetes management routine. However, when starting out in a sport or beginning a new season, more frequent testing is essential. This may mean testing around meal times (before and after) as well as before, during (if possible), and after exercise. There are no rules as to how best to do this, however regular testing provides a clearer picture of how your body responds to exercise. Ultimately, this will allow you to determine the impact of a variety of factors including pre-exercise nutritional status, insulin regimen, insulin injection site, and nature of the exercise on blood glucose control.

Insulin Type And Dose

Seek advice from your diabetes specialist about what insulin regimen (for example, insulin pump or injections) is likely to work for you and how to adjust your insulin according to blood glucose readings and the nature of the exercise you perform. Recording information about how much insulin and what type of insulin you use will provide a basis from which you can progressively alter your regimen according to your exercise demands.

Food Record

A sports dietitian can help you to assess your food diary and see if there are ways to improve your sports performance by modifying your dietary intake.

Energy Levels

This factor relates to how you felt during training. Did you feel tired, lethargic, or full of energy? This may help explain your exercise performance and assist you in monitoring whether you are recovering adequately between exercise sessions.

Initially, it may seem there is a lot of information to be collected. However, collecting detailed information will allow you to identify problem areas and take steps to rectify them. It is beneficial to record the information even when things are going well so you can reflect back on successful strategies in the not so good times. You can use your own codes and very short descriptions to reduce the amount of time required to fill out your diary.

Your diary can be shown to your sports physician, dietitian, diabetes specialist or coach. This network of specialists can help you achieve your sporting goals while managing your diabetes. Not only are they objective, they may also have some great ideas and offer support in the good and bad times.

Chapter 44

Driving When You Have Diabetes

For most people, driving represents freedom, control, and competence. Driving enables most people to get to the places they want or need to go. For many people, driving is important economically—some drive as part of their job or to get to and from work.

Driving is a complex skill. Our ability to drive safely can be affected by changes in our physical, emotional, and mental condition. This chapter will give you the information you need to talk to your health care team about driving and diabetes.

How can having diabetes affect my driving?

In the short term, diabetes can make your blood glucose (sugar) levels too high or too low. As a result, diabetes can make you:

- Feel sleepy or dizzy.

- Feel confused.

- Have blurred vision.

- Lose consciousness or have a seizure.

About This Chapter: Excerpted from "Driving When You Have Diabetes," November 2003, National Highway Traffic Safety Administration, U.S. Department of Transportation.

In the long run, diabetes can lead to problems that affect driving. Diabetes may cause nerve damage in your hands, legs and feet, or eyes. In some cases, diabetes can cause blindness or lead to amputation.

Can I still drive with diabetes?

Yes, people with diabetes are able to drive unless they are limited by certain complications of diabetes. These include severe low blood glucose levels or vision problems. If you are experiencing diabetes-related complications, you should work closely with your diabetes health care team to find out if diabetes affects your ability to drive. If it does, discuss if there are actions you can take to continue to drive safely.

What can I do to ensure that I can drive safely with diabetes?

Insulin and some oral medications can cause blood glucose levels to become dangerously low (hypoglycemia). Do not drive if your blood glucose level is too low. If you do, you might not be able to make good choices, focus on your driving, or control your car. Your health care team can help you determine when you should check your blood glucose level before driving and how often you should check while driving.

If your glucose level is low, eat a snack that contains a fast-acting sugar such as juice, soda with sugar (not diet), hard candy, or glucose tablets. Wait 15 minutes then check your blood glucose again. Treat again as needed. Once your glucose level has risen to your target range, eat a more substantial snack or meal containing protein. Do not continue driving until your blood glucose level has improved.

Most people with diabetes experience warning signs of a low blood glucose level. However, if you experience hypoglycemia without advance warning, you should not drive. Talk to your health care team about how glycemic awareness training might help you sense the beginning stages of hypoglycemia.

In extreme situations, high blood glucose levels (hyperglycemia) also may affect driving. Talk to your health care team if you have a history of very high glucose levels to determine at what point such levels might affect your ability to be a safe driver.

The key to preventing diabetes-related eye problems is good control of blood glucose levels, good blood pressure control, and good eye care. A yearly exam with an eye care professional is essential.

If you are experiencing long-term complications of diabetes such as vision or sensation problems, or if you have had an amputation, your diabetes health care team can refer you to a driving specialist. This specialist can give you on- and off-road tests to see if, and how, your diabetes is affecting your driving. The specialist also may offer training to improve your driving skills. Improving your driving skills could help keep you and others around you safe.

What if I have to cut back or give up driving?

You can keep your independence even if you have to cut back or give up on your driving. It may take planning ahead on your part, but planning will help get you to the places you need to go and to the people you want to see.

Consider:

- Rides with family and friends

- Taxi cabs

- Shuttle buses or vans

- Public buses, trains, and subways

- Walking

☞ Remember!!

Make sure you always carry your blood glucose meter and plenty of snacks (including a quick-acting source of glucose) with you. Pull over as soon as you feel any of the signs of a low blood glucose level. Check your blood glucose.

Chapter 45

Travel Tips For People With Diabetes

As any travel agent or stranded tourist will tell you, planning ahead is the key to a successful trip. And this is particularly true for people with diabetes—a little forethought will take you a long way and help keep you healthy once you are there.

Planning Ahead

Diabetes shouldn't stop you from doing the things you want to do. If you want to travel, and you have diabetes, you must plan ahead carefully. There are many disaster stories such as lost luggage or encountering a hurricane. Traveling can be stressful sometimes—and stress can raise blood glucose levels. Although you can't avoid the odd surprise, preparation before you leave can help you avoid undue stress.

Consider telling your travel agent that you have diabetes and explain some of the particular needs that traveling with diabetes entails. That way, a suitable itinerary can be planned to meet your needs. A missed connection or illness can ruin the best-laid vacation plans.

About This Chapter: Information in this chapter is excerpted from "Travel Tips for People with Diabetes." Reprinted with permission from the Canadian Diabetes Association. To view the complete original text of this article, visit http://www.diabetes.ca. © 2005 Canadian Diabetes Association.

Airport Screening   ✔ Quick Tip

- Notify the screener that you have diabetes and are carrying your supplies with you. The following diabetes-related supplies and equipment are allowed through the checkpoint once they have been screened:
  - Insulin and insulin loaded dispensing products (vials or box of individual vials, jet injectors, pens, infusers, and preloaded syringes)
  - Unlimited number of unused syringes when accompanied by insulin or other injectable medication
  - Lancets, blood glucose meters, blood glucose meter test strips, alcohol swabs, meter-testing solutions
  - Insulin pump and insulin pump supplies (cleaning agents, batteries, plastic tubing, infusion kit, catheter, and needle)
  - Glucagon emergency kit
  - Urine ketone test strips
  - Unlimited number of used syringes when transported in Sharps disposal container or other similar hard-surface container
  - Sharps disposal containers or similar hard-surface disposal container for storing used syringes and test strips
- Insulin in any form or dispenser must be clearly identified.
- If you are concerned or uncomfortable about going through the walk-through metal detector with your insulin pump, notify the screener that you are wearing an insulin pump and would like a full-body pat-down and a visual inspection of your pump instead.
- Advise the screener that the insulin pump cannot be removed because it is inserted with a catheter (needle) under the skin.
- Insulin pumps and supplies must be accompanied by insulin.
- Advise screeners if you are experiencing low blood sugar and are in need of medical assistance.
- You have the option of requesting a visual inspection of your insulin and diabetes associated supplies.

Source: From "Travelers and Consumers: Persons with Diabetes," Transportation Security Administration, U.S. Department of Homeland Security, 2004.

Visit Your Doctor Or Diabetes Educator

It is a good idea to visit your doctor for a checkup several weeks before you leave. Show your itinerary to your health care team and work out plans for your meals and medication, especially if you are traveling through different time zones. Be sure to get any required vaccinations at least four weeks before you travel so you have time to deal with any possible side effects.

Ask for a list of your medications (including the generic names and their dosages) from your pharmacist—particularly oral medications for diabetes and insulin. If you take insulin, record the types of insulin and whether the insulin is short, intermediate or long acting. Photocopy the list and carry one copy with you at all times. Some countries require you to have written documents from your doctor, stating that you are allowed to carry medicines or supplies. Syringes and needles in particular can present a problem when entering some countries.

Identification

Take identification with you that explains your condition in case you are unable to give instructions yourself. Consider getting a MedicAlert® bracelet or necklace that states you have diabetes.

Packing

Divide your medications and diabetes supplies and pack them in more than one place, in case you lose one of your bags. Most importantly, make sure that you have a portion of medications and supplies in your carry-on luggage. Take extra supplies and medication in case of loss, theft, or accidental destruction. Also consider some of the other supplies you may need including treatment for hypoglycemia, food supplies, drinking water, walking shoes, sun block, and medication for nausea and diarrhea.

Planes, Trains, And Automobiles

By Air

Most airlines are more than happy to help with the special needs of their passengers. Airlines usually offer special meals for people with diabetes, but most often the regular airline meals can fit into your meal plan with some careful planning. Always have some appropriate snacks with you in case your flight or in-flight meal is delayed or the meal provided does not have enough carbohydrate. Be aware of time zone changes and schedule your meals and medication accordingly. If you choose to sleep while on board, use a travel alarm clock or ask the flight attendant to wake you at meal or medication time.

If you take insulin, be sure to carry it with you at all times. Manufacturers indicate that, ideally, insulin should not be exposed to x-rays during travel and that it be inspected manually whenever possible. However, the security scanners used at check-in will not normally damage your insulin or blood glucose meter. If baggage remains in the path of the x-ray for longer than normal, or if the baggage is repeatedly x-rayed, the insulin may lose potency. Insulin is affected by extreme temperatures and should never be stored in the unpressurized baggage area of the aircraft. As always, it is important to inspect your insulin before injecting each dose. If you notice anything unusual about the appearance of your insulin, or notice that your insulin needs are changing, contact your doctor.

Try to do some activity during your journey. Walk around in the terminal before boarding. Consider doing simple stretching exercises in your seat. Move your ankles in circles and raise your legs occasionally.

By Car

Whether you are a driver or a passenger, checking your blood glucose regularly is very important. Check your blood glucose before you leave home and then again every four hours during your journey.

Stop every few hours to stretch your legs and do some physical activity. This will help improve blood circulation.

At the first sign of low blood glucose or hypoglycemia, pull over to the side of the road and take a form of fast-acting sugar such as glucose tablets or fruit juice. Follow this with a longer-acting carbohydrate such as a sandwich. Do not start driving again until the symptoms have disappeared and glucose values have improved. If you take insulin, avoid driving in the time between your injection and your next meal. Limit your driving to a maximum of 12 hours per day, or six hours between any two meals.

Keep your medication, meal, and snack times as regular as possible. You may not always be able to get to a restaurant on time, so bring supplies with you to treat low blood glucose (e.g. glucose tablets, hard candy, or fruit juice or regular pop) in case of traffic jams, car trouble, or wrong directions.

By Sea

Cruise vacations are known for all-you-can-eat buffets. With a wide array of mouth-watering foods available, it's easy to overindulge. Talk to your diabetes educator before you leave about how to fit some of these foods into your meal plan. When possible, obtain a sample menu from the cruise line so you can get an idea of the types of foods served. You can then plan your meals accordingly.

Keep active to compensate for extra food eaten. Cruise ships offer some great activities. Try an aerobics class, go for a swim, or stroll the deck at sunset.

It's a good idea to make the cruise staff aware of your diabetes in case any problems arise. Have all of your medications well documented.

By Foot

A vacation in the great outdoors can make for an excellent retreat from the pressures of everyday life, but there are a few things to consider before you go. Most importantly, there is safety in numbers—avoid going camping or hiking alone. Tell someone where you will be and when you expect to return, so you can be found in case of an emergency. Bring along a first aid kit and if you use insulin, a glucagon emergency kit. Teach your travel companion when and how to use glucagon. For more information about the Glucagon Emergency Kit, talk to your diabetes educator.

The key to enjoying a camping trip is to avoid things that severely alter blood glucose levels. Avoid cuts, bruises, sunburns, blisters, insect bites, and contaminated food or water. Of course, make sure you eat and drink enough to meet your needs—bring extra food, water, medication, and sugar. Store your food where animals and bears cannot reach it. If you are extremely active you may need to decrease your diabetes medication, so be sure to discuss this with your diabetes educator or physician.

Insulin Storage And Use

Insulin must be stored properly, as it will spoil if left in temperatures that are too hot or too cold. Insulin retains its potency at room temperature for thirty days.

If you are traveling in hot temperatures, store your insulin in an insulated bag or cooled thermos. In extremely hot conditions, you can freeze water in plastic bottles and keep these in your insulated bag along with your insulin and food supplies. When melted, the water can then serve as drinking water.

If you are skiing, camping, or working in a cold climate, keep your insulin close to your body or an insulated bag to keep it from freezing.

If your trip is short, you may want to keep your needles and sharps and dispose of them on your return home. For longer trips, you can purchase small containers that store or disintegrate needles and syringes.

If you use insulin pens, take a spare one with you. Also, pack some syringes as they can be used in an emergency to withdraw insulin from an insulin cartridge. Remember not to insert air into the cartridge when doing so.

Keeping Blood Glucose Levels Under Control

While on vacation, test your blood glucose frequently. Regular testing is the only way of knowing whether or not your blood glucose levels are in their target range. It is a good idea to bring the instruction manual for your meter as well as extra batteries and test strips with you.

Blood tests can be performed under almost any conditions of travel. Carry alcohol swabs or moist towelettes to wipe your fingers prior to testing when necessary. Keep a daily record of injections, medications, and test results. If you have trouble with your blood glucose levels, follow the adjustment guidelines as discussed with your doctor or diabetes educator and/or contact your doctor or diabetes educator or contact a hospital in the area for advice. Be sure to have your documented list of medications handy to help the doctor provide appropriate care.

If you have opted for travel medical insurance, take your documents to the hospital with you. Insulins have different names and are supplied in different strengths in some countries. Make sure that the insulin and syringe concentrations are the same as those you use at home. Consider using your own supplies of medications and syringes in third world countries. Avoid using local syringes if not sterile.

Time Zone Changes For Insulin Users

Long journeys often cross several time zones. A regular 24-hour day can be extended or shortened depending on the direction of travel. Either way, you'll have to adjust your insulin schedule accordingly. Blood glucose control can be upset by a change in time, altered activity, or disturbance of body rhythm and sleep patterns.

While traveling, keeping your blood glucose close to target levels can be a challenge. Here are some guidelines:

• When traveling east, your travel day will be shorter. If you lose more than two hours, you may need to take fewer units of intermediate or long-acting insulin.

• When traveling west, your travel day will be longer. If you gain more than two hours, you may need to take extra units of short-acting insulin and more food.

• You can change the time of your injections and meals by up to two hours in a day without adjusting your insulin dose or your meal plan.

• Follow your usual meal plan as closely as possible.

If you are crossing more than two time zones, you will need to prepare a meal and insulin schedule with your doctor or diabetes educator before you leave.

Time Zone Changes For People Using Oral Medications For Their Diabetes

If the time difference is less than three hours, you can move the time you take your oral medications by one to one-and-a-half hours. If the time difference is more than three hours, ask your doctor or diabetes educator for advice.

✔ Quick Tip
When You're Away From Home

- Follow your meal plan as much as possible when you eat out. Always carry a snack with you in case you have to wait to be served.

- If you're taking a long trip by car, check your blood glucose before driving. Stop and check your blood glucose every few hours. Always carry snacks like fruit, crackers, juice, or soda in the car in case your blood glucose drops too low.

- Ask ahead of time for a diabetes meal if you're traveling by plane. Most airlines serve special meals for people with health needs. Carry food (like crackers or fruit) with you in case meals are late.

- Carry your medicines (insulin, insulin needles, and diabetes pills) and your blood testing supplies with you. Never put them in your checked luggage.

- Ask your health care team how to adjust your medicines, especially your insulin, if you're traveling across time zones.

- Take comfortable, well-fitting shoes on vacation. You'll probably be walking more than usual, so you should take extra care of your feet.

- If you're going to be away for a long time, ask your doctor for a written prescription for your diabetes medicine and the name of a doctor in the place you're going to visit.

- Don't count on buying extra supplies when you're traveling, especially if you're going to another country. Different countries use different kinds of insulin, needles, and pills.

Source: Excerpted from "Your Guide to Diabetes: Type 1 and Type 2," National Diabetes Information Clearinghouse (NDIC), a service of the National Institute of Diabetes and Digestive and Kidney Diseases (NIDDK), National Institutes of Health (NIH), February 2005.

Eating Well Away From Home

It is probably more difficult to follow your meal plan on the road than it is when you're at home, but it can be done with a little extra planning. Fortunately, a typical diabetes meal plan consists of foods that are generally available in most restaurants.

People with diabetes can fit virtually anything into their meal plan, in moderation. Managing your food intake away from home involves estimating appropriate amounts of these foods. It is a good idea to visit a registered dietitian to learn how to estimate serving sizes. It's also important to eat a balanced diet while you're away from home. Try to keep your calorie intake close to your typical level unless you are more active than usual. With the help of a dietitian, you can vary the types of food you eat. For example, you can try different sources of carbohydrate. Monitoring these changes can help you keep your meal plan on track and may help ward off potential problems.

Always have some snacks with you in case your blood glucose level drops or you're unable to eat your next scheduled meal on time. Cheese and crackers, fresh or dried fruit, granola bars, and sandwiches are all healthy choices that are easy to bring along in a carry-on bag, picnic basket, or cooler. Also bring some quick-acting sugar with you, such as glucose tablets or juice.

The Traveler's Checklist

Before you leave, remember to get:

- a medical check-up.
- travel health insurance.
- an identification card and MedicAlert® bracelet or necklace.
- information on the local foods and drinking water.
- a list of your medications.
- a letter from your doctor.
- any needed vaccinations.
- information on local medical facilities or organizations.

Ask your doctor or health care team about:

- illness management.

- hypoglycemia management (glucagon for insulin users).

- adjustments for meals, insulin, and medications in different time zones.

- avoiding illness caused by contaminated food and water.

- tips for adjusting your medication if required.

Your packing list should include:

- an extra supply of insulin or oral medication for diabetes.

- an extra supply of syringes, needles, and an extra insulin pen if used.

- a blood glucose testing kit and record book.

- fast-acting insulin for high blood glucose and ketones if you use insulin.

- fast-acting sugar to treat low blood glucose.

- extra food to cover delayed meals such as a box of cookies or crackers and fruit juice.

- urine ketone testing strips if you use insulin.

- anti-nausea and anti-diarrhea pills.

- pain medication.

- sun block.

- insect repellent.

- large amounts of bottled water, if necessary.

- comfortable walking shoes.

- glucagon if you use insulin.

- telephone numbers of your doctor and diabetes educator.

- supplies for the trip home in case you run into any problems.

Chapter 46

Diabetes At School

You probably spend about 6 hours or more at school each day—more than one third of your waking hours. If you have diabetes, chances are that during that time you'll need to take care of yourself by checking your blood sugar levels or giving yourself an insulin injection. But the bathroom stalls are a far cry from the comfort and privacy of your own home, and you might be worried about how your friends, classmates, and teachers might react to your diabetes. How can you cope with diabetes at school?

Talking To Teachers And School Staff About Diabetes

Communicating with your teachers about your diabetes can definitely make the school day go a little more smoothly. Your teachers may not know a lot about diabetes, so this is your chance to turn the tables and teach them! You or a parent will probably need to inform your teachers (and other staff members, like your coach, school nurse, or school counselor) about your diabetes and how you'll need to take care of it during the school day. There are a few ways to do this:

About This Chapter: Information in this chapter is from "School and Diabetes." This information was provided by TeensHealth, one of the largest resources online for medically reviewed health information written for parents, kids, and teens. For more articles like this one, visit www.TeensHealth.org, or www.KidsHealth.org. © 2005 The Nemours Center for Children's Health Media, a division of The Nemours Foundation.

Give your teacher, school nurse, and principal's office a copy of your diabetes management plan. This plan talks about what you will need to do during the school day, like test your blood sugar, give yourself injections, or eat lunch at a certain time each day. When your teachers know what needs to be done, they can schedule time into the school day. Your diabetes management plan also contains contact info for your doctors and diabetes health care team, so the school will know how to get in touch if you're sick.

Set up a meeting. If your school already knows about your diabetes and you just want to tell your classroom teachers, you could ask to meet your teacher before or after class to talk about what you might need to do during class, like visit the bathroom to test your blood glucose levels. Perhaps you can agree with your teacher that you can just leave class to use the bathroom or visit the nurse without drawing extra attention to yourself.

If a teacher knows you have diabetes, he or she can also be on the lookout for symptoms of diabetes problems and can call for medical help if you need it. Teachers are busy, so you might need to remind them once in a while that you need to do certain things to take care of your diabetes or that you'll be out for a doctor appointment.

In addition to telling your teachers about your diabetes, it's also a good idea to get to know your school nurse. At some schools, people with diabetes need to get diabetes medicines or test blood sugar levels in the nurse's office.

Write a note. If you feel uncomfortable talking to teachers or school staff about your diabetes, you could write a note or letter instead that goes over what you'll need to do to take care of your diabetes.

In some cases, your school might even work with you and your parents to create a special plan that describes the ways they'll accommodate your diabetes at school. This may involve letting you eat lunch a little early or having a school nurse on site to help you with insulin injections, if you need it.

☞ **Remember!!**
If you have a substitute teacher, let him or her know that you have diabetes and may need to do things like go to the bathroom or get a snack.

Talking To Friends And Classmates About Diabetes

As far as friends and classmates go, it's your call whether you tell them about your diabetes. If friends and classmates know, you don't have to worry what they think when they see you doing things to take care of your diabetes— like giving yourself an insulin injection or checking your blood sugar level. And if you've had diabetes for a while, telling your friends can be a huge relief because you don't have to make up excuses for taking time out to have a snack or go to the bathroom anymore.

Some people will tease anyone who is the slightest bit different from anyone else. Diabetes makes you a little different, so someone might tease you about it. If this happens to you, you're definitely not alone. In one recent study, researchers found that one in three kids and teens with problems like diabetes had to deal with bullying.

What can you do when people tease you? Your friends can be helpful here. For instance, they could say: "Knock it off. Diabetes is no big deal." Ignoring the bully is also a good strategy—bullies thrive on the reaction they get, and if you walk away, you're telling the bully that you just don't care. Sooner or later the bully will probably get bored with trying to bother you. Walk tall and hold your head high. Using this type of body language sends a message that you're not vulnerable. It may also help to talk to a guidance counselor, teacher, or friend—anyone who can give you the support you need. Talking can be a good outlet for the fears and frustrations that can build when you're being bullied.

However you choose to handle teasing or telling your friends, don't try to hide your condition by avoiding treatment or by eating foods that aren't on your meal plan—it'll just make you feel worse and may make you stand out even more.

Taking Care of Diabetes at School

Most of the things you need to take care of your diabetes at home, you'll also need to have at school. It's easy to forget things in the rush to get ready in the morning, so you could try packing your diabetes stuff, like medication, testing supplies, lunch, snacks, water, and your medical identification necklace or bracelet, the night before school.

✔ **Quick Tip**
It's helpful to keep a copy of your diabetes management plan with you all the time—like in your purse, backpack, locker, or car—so you have it for easy reference.

If you run into any diabetes problems at school or you start having symptoms of hypoglycemia or hyperglycemia, do what your plan says you should do, like having a snack or checking your blood glucose levels. (Some teachers don't allow you to eat in class, so be sure your teacher knows what's going on.)

Another part of taking care of diabetes at school is knowing who can help you if you have a question or health emergency. If the school nurse isn't in, is there someone else who can help? Should you call your doctor or your parent? Which kinds of problems can wait until after school and which ones should you handle right away? Talk these things over with your parents, doctor, and someone from school. Write down what you should do and whom you should go to and keep this information with your management plan. Knowing what to do can help you feel more confident if you do have a problem at school.

Chapter 47

Getting Ready For College When You Have Diabetes

Maybe you have been preparing for this, or maybe it sneaked up on you all of a sudden: You have graduated high school and are preparing to start college. You feel proud and excited to be taking this big step toward adulthood, yet you may also be feeling a little anxious.

Most graduating seniors and their parents share mixed feelings of apprehension and excitement before college begins, but teens with diabetes and their parents often have some added concerns. Since the college-bound student will soon have full responsibility for his day-to-day diabetes care, both student and parents want to feel confident that the student can handle his diabetes on his own and fit his self-care routine into college life.

This chapter offers tips and suggestions on making the transition from high school to college easier on the whole family. By creating a plan of action, parents and young adults can lighten their anxiety and be ready for this important period of growth and change.

About This Chapter: Information in this chapter is excerpted from "Getting Ready for College." Reprinted with permission from Diabetes Self-Management. Copyright © 2002 R.A. Rapaport Publishing, Inc. For subscription information, call (800) 234-0923 or visit www.diabetesselfmanagement.com.

Leaving The Nest

Although having full responsibility for diabetes care may seem daunting at first, young adults can, and do, successfully manage their diabetes and thrive in college on their own. It helps a lot, however, if the student is already handling the bulk of care before he leaves home.

From experience, you know that managing diabetes is a balancing act. Not only is it necessary to balance food with activity and insulin, but your family has also balanced the responsibilities for your diabetes care. Ideally, the process of shifting more diabetes care responsibility to you happened gradually as you progressed through high school. Over time, you probably began monitoring your own blood sugar, learning how to determine the amounts of insulin you need to take, and balancing meals and exercise. Usually during high school, parents still need to remind their son or daughter to monitor regularly, take insulin, or carry supplies. In college, however, the student is on his own to remember and carry out diabetes care.

If a teenager is not handling most of his diabetes responsibilities prior to high school graduation, a good time for him to start is during the summer months before the fall college semester begins. This way he is able to have responsibility for care while he still has the safety net of parents in place.

Despite their worries, most parents find that college students manage their diabetes quite well on their own. During semester breaks, parents are often pleasantly surprised by the growth and development that has happened while their son or daughter was away. The teenager they may have struggled with in high school usually grows nicely into adulthood during his time away at college. Taking an interest in diabetes often goes along with this maturity.

Keeping Up With Supplies

As surprising as it may seem to some college freshmen, diabetes supplies will not magically appear in their dormitory room the way they may have at home. Keeping up with supplies is important to avoid last-minute runs to the pharmacy. At college, running out of supplies can be a big problem if the pharmacy is far from the campus and parents are not around to pick up supplies in a pinch.

✔ **Quick Tip**

Before you leave for college, make sure you know how to communicate with your health care providers and educators while you are away. Most likely you will have access to e-mail or to a fax machine. However, if continuing communication with your health team at home will be difficult, you may need to start a new team in your college environment.

Parents should help their teen develop a plan for keeping up with supplies. When they first arrive on campus, parents and student may want to establish a relationship with the local pharmacy, just as they have done at home, so the student knows where prescriptions can be dropped off and how to restock when he needs supplies.

Another way to handle supplies is through a mail-order pharmacy service. Supplies can be delivered directly to the student or sent home so that parents can keep track of orders and payment. Mail-order services usually distribute supplies in three-month increments, eliminating monthly visits to the pharmacy for refills. However, most mail-order pharmacies request notification two weeks prior to the actual date of delivery. Noting reorder dates on the calendar can help you keep track of when to call for refills. If you plan to have supplies delivered to your home at the start of the fall college semester, your reordering schedule should roughly coincide with semester breaks. This will allow you to restock your supplies while at home on visits.

Students should be responsible for keeping up with their supplies or at least notifying parents when they are running low. Dealing with insurance issues and completing the paperwork, however, is something that parents may want to continue to handle to guarantee insurance coverage.

Storing and disposing of supplies safely is important, since casually leaving needles or lancets around can be dangerous. Students will need to work out an arrangement with roommates on where diabetes equipment should be stored in the dormitory room, apartment, or fraternity house.

Students should check with the campus health center to find out how to dispose of sharps (needles and lancets) and syringes. (Loose lancets, needles, and syringes should never be thrown in the trash or in a recycling bin.)

Different campuses may have different regulations. Some colleges may require the student to use a sharps container, while others may say it's OK to use a coffee can or detergent bottle with a secure lid. Likewise, some campuses may want the student to drop off full containers at the health center; while others may allow the student to tape the container shut and throw it in the regular trash.

Dealing With Highs And Lows

Since college living is altogether different from living at home, your blood glucose levels are likely to vary until you adjust to your new surroundings. Don't be overly upset about it; this readjustment happens at first to almost everyone who leaves home.

✔ **Quick Tip**
A convenient way for students to order their diabetes supplies is online. Internet access is readily available on most campuses, and many pharmacies and mail-order houses have Web sites that are set up for online orders. However, it is a good idea to keep copies of written prescriptions at school so the student can go to a local pharmacy and get supplies if there is a problem with delivery of his online order.

The day-to-day variation of class schedules, meal times, and stress and activity levels will influence your diabetes control. Classes may be scheduled during morning hours one day and not until the afternoon the next. Consequently, you may be eating breakfast and taking insulin at 6 a.m. one day and not until 11 a.m. the next. This type of variation will affect your blood sugar level.

Psychological stress can take its toll, too. Being away from home is easy for some and hard for others. Many students get homesick, especially if this is their first time away. The stress of adjustment to college life along with all of the other changes can make moods swing and blood sugar control go haywire.

If your blood sugar level is bouncing wildly from day to day, look at patterns to determine what is making it high or low. Maybe the cafeteria pizza has a bigger effect on your blood glucose than the pizza you ate at home. Maybe low blood sugar is simply the result of the extra walking or biking that you are doing to get from one end of campus to the other. The old regimen from home simply may not work at college.

Here are some blood sugar control rules of thumb for the student to keep in mind as he finds his way:

- Depending on the type of insulin used, there should be no more than four hours between meals and snacks.

- If a student is pulling an all-nighter, he should eat one carbohydrate choice (15 grams of carbohydrate) for every two hours he is awake after his normal bedtime snack.

> ☞ **Remember!!**
>
> It is especially important for you to wear medical identification while at college in case of an emergency. You are new to the college community, and most people will not know about your diabetes. You could end up in a situation where low blood sugar is mistaken for drug or alcohol abuse, which could be dangerous as well as embarrassing.

- Always be prepared to treat hypoglycemia by carrying a source of carbohydrate at all times.

- Keep hypoglycemia treatment options in the dorm room at all times.

For safety reasons, you should inform at least some of your new friends at college about your diabetes and about how to spot and treat hypoglycemia. It's important that you describe your typical symptoms of low blood sugar so they won't be misinterpreted. If your friends know that you become irritable and grumpy when your blood glucose level is low, for example, they will be more likely to understand and help.

Having an informed roommate or buddy could also be a potential life-saver. Although emergencies are unlikely, you should be prepared for them. Even if you have never needed glucagon to treat very low blood sugar, you should ask key people to learn how to use glucagon, just in case.

A Change In The Menu

Another challenging aspect of college life, particularly for a freshman, is adapting to cafeteria food. Although most students are familiar with school menus, eating cafeteria food for every meal can wreak havoc on blood sugar levels.

Weight gain and high blood glucose can develop because of the high-fat and high-carbohydrate choices offered by cafeterias. However, many college cafeterias have made a concerted effort to offer a variety of meal choices,

including healthier options such as salads, baked entrees, and fruits and vegetables. Nonetheless, making appropriate meal choices can be challenging
when you have ample availability of food and no adult looking over your
shoulder. Away from home and the close supervision of parents, some freshmen find it easy to throw their meal plan out the window. This can be frustrating for parents, but ultimately it's up to the student to learn from his
mistakes and control what he eats.

To help the young adults handle the challenge of eating at college, parents and student may want to make an appointment with his dietitian prior
to the start of the fall semester to update his meal plan and review exchanges
and carbohydrate counting.

Most campuses allow students to rent or purchase a refrigerator and/or
microwave for their room. You may want to look into this so you can store
some healthy alternatives if the cafeteria menu doesn't suit your meal plan.

Educating Friends And Teachers

Deciding who in the college community should know about your diabetes is an individual choice. If your family has lived in the same community
throughout high school, you probably have a group of key people—friends,
neighbors, school staff, and coaches—who know about your diabetes. But
going away to school opens up a whole new world, along with a fresh group
of friends and acquaintances. You will again need to decide whom to inform
about your diabetes.

Important people to tell are roommates and resident assistants. These
people need to understand what diabetes is and, most important, understand
the signs, symptoms, and treatment of hypoglycemia. They will also need to be
told that diabetes supplies, such as needles and lancets, will be kept in the room.

Other people who should know are friends you will be spending a lot of
time with. You will probably find that most people are interested and supportive if you are frank and honest with them. If you have had negative
experiences in the past in telling friends, keep in mind that you were probably dealing with younger, less mature individuals. Typically, fellow college
students will be receptive and eager to help.

It is very important for college athletes with diabetes to educate coaches and teammates about diabetes, especially on the treatment of hypoglycemia. Sharing diabetes information with professors is probably not necessary unless the professor has specific rules about eating in the classroom. If this is the case, it would be a good idea to let the professor know that it may be necessary to eat in case of hypoglycemia.

The school's health center should also be informed about your health history and current diabetes regimen. Learning where the health center is located is one of the first things you should do. Parents and the student should also find out how health services are provided on campus and if facilities like hospitals and emergency rooms are accessible.

Drugs And Drinking

It is likely you will be exposed to alcohol, drugs, and smoking on campus, so it is important to address these issues before you leave home. Not only are drugs such as marijuana and cocaine illegal, they also can cause emotional, physical, and psychological problems. If you add diabetes to the mix, it can make matters worse.

While smoking cigarettes may seem less dangerous than using illicit drugs, smoking is the leading preventable cause of death in the United States today. In addition to the long-term health consequences of smoking, such as lung cancer, high blood pressure, heart disease, and stroke, in the short term, smoking reduces teens' lung capacity and rate of lung growth, hampers sports performance, increases the resting heart rate, and causes respiratory problems. Teens who smoke are also much more likely than nonsmokers to use alcohol and other drugs.

Many drugs, including cigarettes, affect appetite, causing the user to either overeat or undereat. For a person with diabetes, an alteration in appetite can greatly affect blood glucose level. Drugs can also change the user's mental state, which can result in the person forgetting to eat or, in the case of a person with diabetes, to check his blood sugar level or take his insulin.

The same problem can occur with alcohol use. Even though in most states alcohol is legal for people 21 and over, it is still considered a drug. Alcohol can cause confusion, forgetfulness, and changes in blood sugar level. If you decide to drink alcohol, you should be aware of some precautions to take because drinking too much or drinking at the wrong time of day can be dangerous for someone who has diabetes. It is a good idea for parents to sit down and talk with their young adult before he leaves for college so that he has a better understanding of what could happen to him if he drinks and to formulate some guidelines for safe experimentation.

Alcohol lowers blood sugar level. This effect can last anywhere from six to 36 hours after the last drink, depending on the amount of alcohol consumed. Since alcohol can also mask the symptoms of hypoglycemia, anyone with diabetes should check his blood sugar level during and after drinking alcohol to make sure he is not hypoglycemic. To counter the blood-glucose-lowering effect of alcohol, it helps to eat while drinking. And of course, drinking in moderation is safer for everyone.

Choosing Adult Diabetes Care

Continued diabetes care and follow-up is very important during the young adult years. Many pediatricians and pediatric diabetes centers will provide continued follow-up care for their patients throughout college. Most, however, will refer the young person to adult services once he graduates college.

Whether a student continues diabetes care with a pediatrician or pediatric endocrinologist throughout college is an individual choice. Some feel that the young college student is dealing with so many changes that adjusting to new health-care services simply complicates matters. Others think that the transition to college is a good time to change to adult care services. The decision should be discussed with the doctor and be based on what is most comfortable for the student.

It is very important, however, that the student have a physician available near to the campus community in case of an emergency, illness, or any other health care issue that arises during the year. If the campus health center does not seem to meet your needs, a local physician can offer more individual or comprehensive care.

Routine visits to your usual health-care provider can be scheduled for college breaks to eliminate the need for special trips home. With busy college schedules, it is easy to forget or neglect routine checkups. At this time probably more than ever, keeping up with diabetes care is extremely important.

As your family takes this important step forward, it is wise to schedule an education appointment with a diabetes educator before you go off to college. Often, diabetes education is directed to the parents, especially if the teen was diagnosed with diabetes at a young age. Now is a good time for a refresher course that includes special emphasis on how to fit good diabetes care into campus life.

Chapter 48

Education And Your Legal Rights As A Student With Diabetes

The Laws

The right of children with diabetes to care for their diabetes at school is based on the Section 504 of the Rehabilitation Act of 1973, the Americans with Disabilities Act, and the Individuals with Disability Education Act (IDEA). These laws provide protection against discrimination for children with disabilities, including diabetes, in any program or activity receiving federal financial assistance. This includes all public schools and day care centers and those private schools and centers that receive federal funds.

There seems to be a lot of confusion regarding the differences between a 504 and Individualized Education Plan (IEP). To put it simply, a 504 plan is a plan designed to deal with medical issues, such as diabetes, while an IEP is a plan designed to deal with educational challenges or special needs that need not be related to a medical treatment plan. A 504 would contain instructions, for example, for blood glucose monitoring, while an IEP would include instructions for additional reading education, should it be needed.

About This Chapter: "The Law, Schools, and Your Child with Diabetes," © 2004 Children with Diabetes and Diabetes 123. All rights reserved. Reprinted with permission. For additional information, visit http://www.childrenwithdiabetes.com.

Children with diabetes use a 504 plan for accommodations related to diabetes and need not have an IEP unless they have special academic needs.

- **Section 504 of the Rehabilitation Act of 1973**—According to this law, parents of qualifying children have the right to develop a Section 504 plan with their child's school. To qualify for protection under Section 504, a child must have a record of such impairment, or be regarded as having such impairment. Schools can lose federal funding if they do not comply with this law. Parents can use these laws to ensure that, while at school, their children with diabetes can fully participate in all school activities, while at the same time caring for their medical needs. This means that the school cannot refuse to allow a child with a 504 to be on the honor roll, deny credit to a student whose absenteeism is related to diabetes, refuse to administer medication (a school cannot require parents to waive liability as a condition of giving medicine), and determine sports/extracurricular participation without regard to the student's diabetes. Any school that receives federal funding must comply with IDEA and Section 504 laws. A child need not require special education to be protected.

- **The Americans with Disabilities Act**—This law prohibits all schools and day care centers, except those run by religious organizations, from discriminating against children with disabilities, including diabetes. Protection under this law is the same as that for Section 504.

- **Individuals with Disabilities Education Act (IDEA)**—IDEA mandates the federal government to provide funding to education agencies, state and local, to provide free and appropriate education to qualifying students with disabilities. This includes children who have diabetes. As with the other two laws, you must show that diabetes can, at times, adversely affect educational performance. The school is then required to develop an Individualized Education Plan (IEP) to accommodate the child's needs.

> **✤ It's A Fact!!**
>
> A 504 plan is a plan designed to deal with medical issues, such as diabetes, while an IEP is a plan designed to deal with educational challenges or special needs that need not be related to a medical treatment plan.

• **State Regulations**—Some states have enacted additional legislation to protect children with disabilities. Contact your state legislature for further information.

What This Means

Any educational facility, school or daycare center, which receives federal funding, cannot discriminate in the admission, educational process, or treatment of a student who has diabetes. Provided that the presence of diabetes has been disclosed and verified, and that the student/parents have requested reasonable accommodations, the educational facility is required by law to make the approved modifications which allow the child with diabetes to fully participate and benefit from all school activities and programs.

The student/parents are not required to assume responsibility for the provision of needed accommodations. However, the school can refuse to grant a request for an accommodation that is not specifically documented. School personnel do not have the right to confidential medical information. They need only to know what needs to be done to guarantee equal opportunity for the student. Any individual member of school staff who fails to comply with the approved medical and education plan can be held personally liable.

Responsibilities

• **Student or Parents**

1. In a timely manner, identify that the child has diabetes.

2. Provide recent documentation that the child has diabetes.

3. In writing, request needed accommodations.

4. Request a meeting to discuss 504 Plan and IEP.

• **School Personnel**

1. Provide written assurance of nondiscrimination.

2. Provide notice of nondiscrimination in admission or access to its programs or activities. Notice must be included in a student/parent handbook.

♣ It's A Fact!!
School Bill Of Rights For Children With Diabetes

Children with diabetes require medical care to remain healthy. The need for medical care does not end while the child is at school. Thus, while at school, each child with diabetes must be allowed to:

1. Do blood sugar checks.

2. Treat hypoglycemia with emergency sugar.

3. Inject insulin when necessary.

4. Eat snacks when necessary.

5. Eat lunch at an appropriate time and have enough time to finish the meal.

6. Have free and unrestricted access to water and the bathroom.

7. Participate fully in physical education (gym class) and other extracurricular activities, including field trips.

Taking Action Against Discrimination

If you are faced with a school that does not comply with the School Bill of Rights for Children with Diabetes, you should first educate the school administration. Make sure they understand the laws and the child's needs.

Schools that still refuse to cooperate should be advised that you are requesting preparation of an Individualized Education Program (IEP) and a Section 504 Accommodation. At this point, the school must meet with you to negotiate the special services that the child requires. You should begin with the entire list of services in the School Bill of Rights for Children with Diabetes.

If your school still refuses to comply with the School Bill of Rights for Children with Diabetes, you should file a complaint with your state's department of education. This is the first step in the process of litigation against your school system.

The child has a right to care for his or her diabetes at school. The scientific data are clear on the value of maintaining glycemic control. Since there is no break from diabetes, there can be no break from the need to care for it. Time spent at school is no exception.

Source: "School Bill of Rights for Children with Diabetes," © 2002 Children with Diabetes and Diabetes 123. All rights reserved. Reprinted with permission. For additional information, visit http://www.childrenwithdiabetes.com.

3. Designate an employee to coordinate compliance.

4. Cooperate in providing authorized accommodations.

5. Request physician's specific recommendations of needed accommodations.

6. Request a meeting to discuss 504 Plan and IEP.

7. Provide grievance procedures to resolve complaints.

What To Include In A 504 Plan

1. Medication procedures and dosages (e.g. insulin administration prior to meals, etc.) You will want to note if the child is capable of deciding that amount to be given or provide an alternative such as calling a parent or using a chart to determine amount to be given.

2. Blood glucose testing procedures (when, where, etc.). The school does have the right to not allow blood glucose testing in the classroom. However, if you can demonstrate that this procedure will not endanger others (i.e., materials will be disposed of at home and not at school), your school may allow the child to check in a secure area in the classroom.

3. Procedures for treatment of hyper and hypoglycemia.

4. Precautions to be taken before physical activity.

5. Guidelines for meals, snacks, special treats, and parties.

6. Contact information for medical assistance (as needed) and parents.

What To Include In An IEP

1. The need for repeat of information. Sometimes, if a child has had an insulin reaction or extremely high blood sugar, that child may not be able to concentrate and need additional assistance.

2. The child with diabetes may need to be allowed to take make-up tests if that student has had an insulin reaction or severe hyperglycemia during an exam.

3. Flexibility in attendance requirements in case of health-related absences including physician visits (e.g., allowing students to be on honor roll and qualify for awards, etc.).

4. Permission to leave class to use restroom as needed.

5. Provision of adequate time for taking medication, checking blood sugars, and completing meals and snacks.

6. Access to increased fluid intake as needed.

Chapter 49

Diabetes At Work

Get up, get showered, get breakfast, go to school, get to work. You need money; therefore you have a job.

But you also have diabetes. Maybe you had diabetes before you started working. Maybe you've been working for years and have been diagnosed recently. Either way, you have to care for your diabetes while you're at work. Here are some tips for merging your diabetes care with your career.

Decide Who To Tell

Should you share your diabetes status with your co-workers? All things being equal, it might be in your best interest to let a few trusted co-workers or your boss know.

"I do recommend that a few people know about your diabetes, just for your own safety," says Terry Lumber, RN, MSN, CDE, BCADM, a diabetes clinical nurse specialist at Inova Fair Oaks Hospital in Fairfax, Va. "It helps to think ahead and prepare for how you're going to tell people, and whom."

However, it's possible that you don't feel comfortable letting other people know about your diabetes. In the end, it's up to you.

"It depends on the situation and the person, and it depends on the office," says Kris Smith, RN, MSN, CDE, diabetes educator at the Diabetes and Metabolic Diseases Center in Wilmington, Del. "It depends on whether you are comfortable sharing your diabetes status with your co-workers."

She suggests that you consider how often you have low blood sugars. If you have them frequently, it may help to have an ally at work who knows what the signs are and how to help you. Also, if there's a company nurse at your work site, he or she would be a good person to tell.

> ✔ **Quick Tip**
> **Wear Medical Identification Jewelry**
>
> Whether or not you tell your co-workers about your diabetes, you should wear some form of medical alert jewelry or identification. If you ever need medical assistance at work, the emergency medical personnel will know you have diabetes.

Give Your Co-Workers A Chance

Don't just assume that your boss won't accommodate you, or that your co-workers won't be helpful. Give them a chance to grasp what diabetes is and understand how they can help you, particularly if you've been diagnosed since starting your current job. Diabetes may be as new to them as it is to you.

"If there is a problem that needs to be fixed, don't get mad," says Kathleen Stanley, CDE, CN, RD, LD, MSEd, diabetes education program coordinator and instructor at Central Baptist Hospital in Lexington, Ky. "Give your supervisor a chance to fix it. Sometimes people get upset and go right to the highest person on the chain, and it turns out their immediate supervisor never knew about the diabetes. Recognize your lines of authority. Most supervisors are willing to work with their employees to help them do their jobs."

Don't assume the worst about people, either, says Lumber. For instance, you may be at lunch with your co-workers and they might glance at you sideways if you order dessert. They might even ask you if you should be having dessert at all. Use the opportunity to educate them.

"Acknowledge that people are trying to be helpful, but maybe they blurt things out the wrong way," Lumber says. "Explain that you know how to handle your diet, and that you have a plan and this is part of your plan. Instead of getting angry, tell them how they can help you. Once people understand, they tend to back off, particularly co-workers."

Get It In Writing

If necessary, get a doctor's note, says Stanley. "It may help to get a medical statement from your doctor saying what your diabetes care needs are. Present it to your company nurse or human resources department, and make sure your supervisor gets a copy. Most employers are willing to meet the needs outlined in the letter, and the Americans with Disabilities Act is there to help ensure that they do."

Whether or not you tell your co-workers about your diabetes, there are steps you must take for your personal well being.

Be Your Own Advocate

Your local hospital or diabetes center may offer programs through which diabetes educators can come to your workplace and explain to your human resources department, supervisors, or co-workers what diabetes is and how they can make the workplace more diabetes-friendly. See if your employer is willing to host such a program.

But don't just look at the big picture. For instance, if the company vending machines are filled with chips, candy, and cookies, talk to your human resources department about stocking more nutritious snacks instead. Ask about nuts, fruit, low-fat crackers, and yogurt.

Don't Abuse The System

Unfortunately, there are people who claim extensive health challenges and reap disability benefits their situation may not warrant, says Stanley.

♣ It's A Fact!!
Diabetes And Employment—Questions And Answers

What are the potential difficulties with regard to employment?

It is important that you disclose your diabetes if required to do so on an employment application. There is no reason why people with diabetes should not have equal access to job opportunities. Difficulties may be encountered due to treatment with insulin or due to complications of diabetes. Treatment with insulin, even with careful monitoring, carries a risk of hypoglycemia, which may be considered to be unacceptable to certain employers. Complications such as retinopathy with visual impairment, or angina may turn out to be an obstacle to securing the job you want. Your prospective employer may also consider the possibility of your job being hazardous to your health.

What factors will my doctor and employer take into consideration?

Some or all of the following may be taken into account when assessing the situation.

- Is your diabetes stable (well controlled)?

- Have you had any disabling hypos, that is—hypoglycemia requiring assistance from another person?

- Have you normal awareness of hypoglycemia?

Do you have any evidence of severe complications, such as advanced retinopathy, kidney disease, peripheral neuropathy, or circulatory problems?

Are there any jobs which are denied to people on insulin?

Yes. Unfortunately being on insulin might preclude you from taking up the following opportunities:

- Driving buses and taxis

- Armed forces

- Fire service

- Ambulance service

- Prison service

- Airline pilots and airline cabin crew

- Air traffic control

- Offshore work, for example—on oil rigs and ships

This list is by no means exhaustive. You may feel (justifiably) that some employers unfairly prevent you from taking a job, which you could safely undertake. Individual cases are best discussed further with your doctor.

What about shift work and diabetes?

Shift work often leads to difficulty with diabetes control, especially for people on insulin. Proper training and self-monitoring are essential.

Frequent changes in daily routine with spells of night duty present problems with working out timing and dosage of insulin injections. If shift work is to be undertaken, shifts from 6:00 a.m. to 10:00 p.m., ideally excluding night duty should be considered.

Why is shift work disruptive?

- Changes to timing of meals

- Variations in level of activity at night

- Variations in levels of stress

- Difficulty in injecting at work

- Timing of periods of "catch-up" sleep (interferes with meals and injections)

Should I change jobs?

Ideally, not. Many employers will now accommodate you within the same organization even if it means a change of role.

What is the ideal job?

- Fixed working hours

- Regular physical activity rather than an overly sedentary desk-bound occupation

- Ability to perform self-monitoring and injections at work

That makes it harder for everyone. It's best to save sick days and disability pay for when you really need them.

Try to schedule your doctor visits for early in the morning or later in the day to be less disruptive of core work hours. Another option is to schedule more than one appointment for the same day. Either way, let your supervisor know well ahead of time that you'll need to take time for the challenge of uncooperative doctor's appointments, and offer to make up the work, says Stanley. "Don't just say, 'I need to do this tomorrow.' Follow your company's leave policy," she says.

She suggests calling your doctor's office the day of your appointment to see if your doctor is on schedule. If your doctor is running late, you can continue to work until you need to go, instead of wasting your time in a waiting room.

Plan Ahead

"The biggest challenge many people with diabetes face is access to meals and breaks," says Lumber. "A little pre-planning is needed more than anything else."

To that end, she suggests having snacks readily available should you need to treat a low. If you work at a desk, keep non-perishable snacks like peanut butter crackers or cans of regular (non-diet) soda in a drawer. If you're on the road a lot, keep non-perishable snacks with you in the car.

However, if you work on a production line or far from where you keep your possessions, it might be best to keep your snack in a pocket or fanny pack. "We encourage people to keep snacks on their person. A locker or car may be too far away, and you might not be able to get to it in time," she says.

Take Your Equipment With You

Keep your blood glucose meter and supplies where you can reach them. Don't leave blood glucose meters or insulin in the car. Extreme temperatures can affect them. Depending on how open you are about your diabetes, you might wish to keep your meter on your desk to remind you to check your blood sugars.

Watch Out For Stress

Stress can wreak havoc on your blood sugars. "If you're having a high-stress workday, your blood sugars may be high," says Rosemary Cobb, RN, BSN, CDE, coordinator of the pregnancy and diabetes program at the Diabetes and Metabolic Diseases Center in Wilmington, Del. "That's the day you want to go for a walk on your lunch hour or make adjustments in your insulin or medication."

Stress can cause either high or low blood sugar. It differs from person to person and sometimes from situation to situation in the same person. Stress may mask symptoms of low blood sugar, or prompt completely different symptoms. Frequent monitoring is your best defense.

Revisit Your Treatment

If you're worried about calling attention to yourself with a vial and syringe, an insulin pen or pump may be more discreet. A pump may be particularly helpful if you have an erratic work schedule or do shift work, because you can store different insulin delivery programs and select the one you need each day. If you have type 2 and take diabetes pills, and you experience low blood sugars at work because of delayed lunches and snacks, it might be time to talk to your doctor about taking a different kind of pill.

Keep Good Diabetes Control

The best thing you can do to remain productive is to stay healthy, says Cobb. "Don't let your diabetes get so far out of control that you're not able to work. If you're eating well, exercising, and controlling your blood sugars, you should have a productive work life."

The payoff here—aside from a job well done—is that if and when you need to take time off for your diabetes care, your boss and co-workers will remember your good track record and be that much more willing to cover for you or help you with scheduling. By communicating with your employer and taking responsibility for your care, you can incorporate your diabetes care into your work life successfully.

The Challenge Of Uncooperative Employers

Ideally, all you'd need to do to ensure that you can properly care for your diabetes at work is ask.

Ideally.

Sometimes, bosses and co-workers just don't get it. Your boss might refuse to allow you to take a regular lunch break, or breaks to check your blood sugars. In that case, your boss would not only be uncooperative, he or she would be violating the Americans with Disabilities Act. The Act requires employers to make "reasonable accommodations" if requested by employees with a disability. Checking your blood sugars and eating regularly fall into that category, as does keeping your supplies nearby.

On the other hand, maybe your boss is willing to accommodate your needs, but your co-workers think it's unfair that you "get to take breaks" or keep a regular schedule when they don't. Under the Act, your boss is not allowed to tell your co-workers about your diabetes (or any other health condition you may have) unless it's on a "need-to-know" basis or unless you give your boss permission to do so. Likewise, without your permission, your boss is not allowed to explain why you are stepping away from your work to have a snack. It may just be easier for you to take control and explain what's going on to your co-workers.

Chapter 50

Dealing With Sick Days

Sick day management is probably one of the most important and trickiest aspects of managing your diabetes. It can also be one of the most frightening. If not properly taken care of, it can most certainly result in being admitted to a hospital for further observation and treatment.

There are many kinds of illnesses that can disrupt your blood glucose control—viral colds or flu, infections, injuries, fever, vomiting, and diarrhea. Emotional stress and surgery can also affect blood glucose level. Learning to manage sick days at home is vital so that you can avoid hospitalization, and it will also make you feel more comfortable until your illness has passed.

When a person with diabetes gets sick, you will notice that blood sugars will often be higher than usual, even if you are eating less food. This is because insulin is often not as effective when you are ill. Also, keep in mind that during your illness the liver is still releasing sugar even when one cannot eat, so your body still needs insulin.

The most common cause for hospitalization among people with diabetes is DKA or diabetes ketoacidosis. The major cause of DKA is usually viral and bacterial infections.

Sick Day Plan

It is vital that you and your diabetes health care team develop a plan for sick days in advance. This plan should tell you how often to measure blood sugar and urine ketones, what medicines to take for what symptoms, and how and what to eat, and even when to call the doctor. You should also compile a sick day emergency kit so that you can have on hand the supplies that you need to manage sick days.

Also, you should attach to your plan a list of phone numbers for your doctor, diabetes educator, and dietitian. Make sure you also know how to reach them at night and on weekends and holidays. Then, when illness strikes, you will be ready.

Quick Guidelines Of Do's And Don'ts

1. Do take your insulin or medication. Always take your insulin or diabetes medication as usual, unless your doctor instructs you differently. Even if you cannot eat anything, your body needs insulin. You might even require additional insulin or medication to manage your diabetes during this period. Check with your doctor before you make any adjustments.

2. Do test your blood sugar every 2 to 4 hours. Get someone to help you if you need it.

3. Do test your urine for ketones every 4 hours.

4. Do drink clear liquids (at least ½ cup every hour), and eat light foods if you can.

5. Do rest. Do not exercise during an illness.

Different illnesses may have a different impact on the diabetes. Generally, conditions with high temperatures cause insulin resistance and increased need for insulin while conditions with low temperatures and vomiting may call for reduced insulin requirements. The insulin requirement during fever is individual, but a rule of thumb is that the insulin requirement increases by 25% per degree of temperature over 37.5°C.

Ketone bodies may be demonstrated in conditions both with high and low blood glucose. In the former situation, a serious lack of insulin exists in the body, and the condition may progress to DKA if extra insulin is not given. In the latter situation, the ketone bodies are "hunger" related and are often associated with low blood glucose values.

In either situation insulin should never be omitted, even if you are unable to eat.

When To Call For Help

Most often than not, a person with diabetes can be effectively managed at home with their own knowledge and some advice from the diabetes team.

There are, however, certain situations in which you should be admitted to the hospital for further observation and treatment:

- You have an obvious infection

- Your illness lasts longer than 2 days

- Persistent vomiting or diarrhea more than 8 hours

- Your blood sugar is over 400 mg in two consecutive tests, and you have moderate to large urine ketones with a blood glucose for more than 8 hours despite adequate treatment

- You feel very ill or experience pain

- You have extreme fatigue, shortness of breath, or dizziness

- Increasing ketone bodies in the urine

- Abdominal pain

👉 **Remember!!**

To put it in simple terms, for sick day management at home you need to do frequent (every 2–4 hours) blood glucose measurements, frequent urine testing for ketone bodies, and be in close contact with the diabetes team for advice.

It is important that the families are taught to react adequately in case of intercurrent illnesses, and the diabetes team should provide the family with written instructions concerning sick day management at home.

Food And Eating

Eating and drinking can be a big problem on sick days. If you can, it's important to stick to your normal meal plan. To keep from getting dehydrated, you should try to drink lots of non-caloric liquids. These are liquids like water and diet soft drinks. It's easy to run low on fluids when you are vomiting or have a fever or diarrhea. Extra fluids will also help flush extra sugar, and sometimes ketones, in your blood.

Your sick day plan should contain a special meal plan in case you can't stick to your normal meal plan. Try to take in your normal number of calories by eating easy-on-the-stomach foods like regular (non-diet) gelatin, crackers, soups, and applesauce.

If even these mild foods are too hard to eat, you may have to stick to drinking liquids that contain carbohydrates. You might try drinking sugared (not diet) soft drinks or other high-carbohydrate liquids such as juice, frozen juice bars, sherbet, pudding, creamed soups, and fruit-flavored yogurt. Broth is also a good choice. 40 to 50 grams of carbohydrate every three to four hours might be a good target to aim for. Check with your doctor to get an individual target range. If you cannot hold down any liquid or solid food you might try dipping your finger in sugar and eating that. This is a good way of getting raw calories when you have insulin in you.

To prepare for sick days, have on hand at home a small stock of these items:

1. **Liquids**

    • Fruit juice: apple, cranberry, grape, grapefruit, orange, pineapple, etc.

    • Sugar-containing beverages: regular 7Up®, gingerale, orange, cola, PEPSI®, etc.

    • Fruit flavored drinks: regular Kool-Aid®, lemonade, Hi-C®, etc.

- Sports drinks: Gatorade®, POWERADE®, etc. (any flavor)

- Tea with honey or brown sugar

- JELL-O®: regular and sugar free

- Popsicles: regular and sugar free

- Broth-type soup: bouillon, chicken noodle soup, Cup-a-Soup®

2. **Solids (when ready)**

- Graham crackers and saltine crackers

- Banana (or other fruit)

- Applesauce

- Bread or toast

- Chicken noodle soup

✎ What's It Mean?

Diabetic Ketoacidosis: An emergency condition in which extremely high blood glucose levels, along with a severe lack of insulin, result in the breakdown of body fat for energy and an accumulation of ketones in the blood and urine. Signs of DKA are nausea and vomiting, stomach pain, fruity breath odor, and rapid breathing. Untreated DKA can lead to coma and death.

Ketone: A chemical produced when there is a shortage of insulin in the blood and the body breaks down body fat for energy. High levels of ketones can lead to diabetic ketoacidosis and coma. Sometimes referred to as ketone bodies.

Ketonuria: A condition occurring when ketones are present in the urine, a warning sign of diabetic ketoacidosis.

Source: "Diabetes Dictionary," National Diabetes Information Clearinghouse (NDIC), a publication of the National Institute of Diabetes and Digestive and Kidney Diseases (NIDDK), National Institutes of Health (NIH), NIH Publication No. 04-3016, November 2003; available at http://diabetes.niddk.nih.gov/dm/pubs/dictionary.

Treating Ketones Yourself

Learning to treat yourself for ketones is probably the single most important aspect of sick day management. It can mean the difference between dealing with your illness or stress in the comforts of your own home or spending days or up to a week in the hospital.

Ketonuria is the appearance of moderate or large ketones in the urine, which can develop into acidosis. Ketonuria and acidosis are due to there not being enough insulin available to meet the body's needs. Acidosis is a very serious and dangerous condition. If left untreated, you could possibly go into a coma and die from it. It is the cause of 85% of hospitalizations of children and adults with diabetes.

The main causes of acidosis are when there is a stress on your body from an illness or surgery, skipping an insulin shot, or there is simply not enough insulin to handle the carbohydrate consumption. With an illness, extra energy may be needed by the body. This cannot be made unless extra insulin is available to make the extra energy from sugar.

How To Test For Ketones

The measurement of urine ketones is quite easy. There are two ways to do this—ketone dipsticks or there are a few glucose meters that also read ketones. For the dipstick method, all that is required is a ketone dipstick to come in contact with your urine. It can either be dipped or passed through a stream of urine. There will be a color chart on the box that the dipstick came in. Just match it up to get your ketone level. Read the directions carefully.

For the meter, you will have to use the ketone calibration strip that comes with your meter. Insert a ketone strip in the meter and draw the blood from a finger as you would for a regular blood glucose test. It's very similar to a regular blood glucose test.

Adding Insulin

It is very important to check with your doctor before trying this very important part of managing your sick days. These are only general guidelines to help you grasp the concept. Every person is different, so the dose of extra insulin varies from person to person, and your doctor will help you decide on a safe dose.

For light to moderate ketones, the extra dose is usually in the range of 5–10% of the total daily dose and is given as Humalog or Regular insulin every two or three hours. For large ketones, 15–20% of the total daily dose (given as Humalog or Regular insulin) is usually given every two or three hours. The blood sugar should be checked before each insulin injection and 1 to 2 hours after each injection.

If the blood sugar drops below 150 mg/dl, it may be necessary to drink something with carbohydrates, like juice, regular soda pop (with sugar), or other sugared drinks to bring the blood sugar back up before giving the next insulin injection. This extra insulin, along with fluids, is being taken to get rid of the ketones in your urine. This dose of extra insulin may seem large, but ketones block the normal sensitivity of the body to insulin.

Although every person is different, these are average dosages that are usually needed to flush ketones from the body and prevent acidosis. This additional Regular/Humalog insulin helps your body use the sugar in the blood and prevents breakdown of fat cells.

Sick Day Emergency Tool Kit

It is recommended that all patients with diabetes should have a diabetes sick day emergency tool kit. There are specific sick day guidelines about fluids, frequency of checking your blood sugar level, and other ideas that you should talk over with your doctor and/or diabetes nurse educator.

Fast Acting Or Regular Insulin For Treating High Blood Sugar

Keep a spare bottle of your Lispro/Humalog or Regular ("R") insulin in your refrigerator for possible use in sick day emergency situations when your sugar levels are high. Your doctor will give you instructions on when and how to use this insulin. Do not use this Lispro/Humalog or "R" insulin except as instructed by your doctor. Lispro/Humalog works a lot faster than Regular to knock down elevated blood sugars, and is preferred for this purpose by most patients.

Glucagon Kit®

This is for treating severe insulin reactions or for small injections to counteract hypoglycemia during spells of vomiting. During severe insulin reactions, it is for use by a family member or friend, if you are unable to take sugar by mouth. You should give your family instructions on when and how to use glucagon. Glucagon does require a prescription.

Compazine® or Phenergan®

These are for treating nausea, by mouth or rectal suppository. Read the directions carefully for each and follow them. These do require a prescription, so ask your doctor for one. These are available as generic versions at lesser cost.

Imodium®

This is for treating diarrhea. Follow the directions carefully. We recommend the capsule version, since the liquid version contains alcohol. Imodium® does not need a prescription.

Sick Day Snacks

You should plan ahead and keep certain items on hand for you to manage your sick days when the situation arises.

Please note that some of the medications listed above are for adults. Ask your doctor what is appropriate. Generic versions of many medications are frequently available, and may be cheaper. Ask your pharmacist. We would recommend the generic versions of all of these, except insulin.

> ✔ **Quick Tip**
> Make a list and give it to your doctor so he/she can help you put together this kit and keep these medications at your home in case they're needed.

Chapter 51

Be Prepared To Handle Diabetes In An Emergency Or Natural Disaster

Proper diabetes care takes a lot of planning. Unexpected events such as floods, tornadoes, earthquakes, and electrical storms make diabetes management more difficult. You can be ready for disasters by storing medical supplies and food supplies in a place where you can easily find them. Plastic or metal boxes help keep your essential items dry.

Medical Supplies

Store enough of the following supplies to last two weeks. Check the expiration dates of your supplies every two or three months and replace as needed.

- Two bottles of each type of your insulins (bottles, pre-filled cartridges, or pre-filled pens). These must be kept in the refrigerator, not in your diabetes kit.

- Two bottles of any other medications you take.

- Syringes and/or pen needles.

- If you use an insulin pump, include: infusion sets, insertion devices, batteries for the pump and remote, and antiseptic wipes.

About This Chapter: Information in this chapter is from "Preparing for Disaster Conditions." Reprinted from http://www.BDDiabetes.com, courtesy of Becton, Dickinson Company, © 2005. All rights reserved.

✔ Quick Tip
Smart Tips For Disaster Conditions

- Always take your insulin as usual.

- All unopened bottled insulin (except Lantus®, which should be stored in a refrigerator or kept below 86°F) can stay at room temperature for 30 days.

- Once an insulin bottle is open, it is good for only 30 days—even if refrigerated.

- Insulin shouldn't be kept in direct sunlight or be exposed to temperatures above 86°F for too long.

- Read the insulin product insert if you have additional questions.

- If you're keeping insulin in a cooler, the temperature shouldn't go below 35°F.

- Before drawing up insulin (or injecting it with a pen), check the bottle or cartridge for frosting or clumps inside of the glass.

- If you find clumps or crystals in your insulin, use another bottle. If this is the only insulin you have left, try to use it. (Note: Depending upon its condition, it may be difficult to draw into your syringe.)

- Syringes and lancets should be kept dry, with the needle shield or cap intact.

- Unless you have no other supplies with which to inject, NEVER reuse your insulin syringes, pen needles, or lancets! If you have no fresh syringes or lancets to use, ONLY reuse your own syringes, pen needles, or lancets. Using someone else's supplies could cause infection or spread disease.

- Alcohol swabs.

- Blood glucose meter and test strips.

- Lancets and lancet device.

- A blood sugar testing diary.

- Urine ketone testing strips.

- Glucose tablets, cans of regular soda, juice, and hard candies.

- Glucagon emergency kit.

- Home sharps container for disposal.

- Prescriptions for diabetes supplies.

- Medication for nausea, vomiting, and diarrhea.

- An insulated bag for your insulin supplies (to protect your supplies if there's a power outage, especially in warm climates).

Food Supplies And Meal Plan

Store the following foods in a place that's dry and easy to reach:

- 1 large unopened box of crackers

- 1 large jar of peanut butter

- 1 small box of powdered milk

- 1 gallon of water per day for at least one week

- 2 packages of cheese and crackers or 1 jar of soft cheese

- 1 package of dry, unsweetened cereal

- 6 cans of sugar-free soda

- 1 six-pack of canned fruit juice or sports drink

- 1 spoon, fork, and knife per person

- disposable cups

- 4 packages of glucose tablets or small hard candies

- several cans of tuna, salmon, chicken, and nuts

- a manual can opener

Try to follow your meal plan as closely as possible and never skip a meal. It's important to avoid getting hungry or overeating, especially in disaster conditions. If you think your running water may be contaminated, boil it for three minutes. If you're not feeling well or run out of medicine and/or food, seek medical attention as soon as possible.

Part Five

Coping With Feelings And Relationships

Chapter 52

The Emotional Challenge Of Diabetes

"I feel embarrassed giving myself shots in front of people. One day I had to give myself an insulin shot in the bathroom at the train station and this guy looked at me like I was doing drugs. That felt humiliating."

"Why do I have to go through this when my friends don't have to follow a meal plan, test their blood sugar levels, or have shots all the time?"

"I worry that I'm a burden on my family. I feel guilty that my dad has to drive me to doctor's appointments and pay for it all."

"I get angry at my mom. I know she worries about me, but she's always nagging me about what I eat and stuff. My kid sister has it easy."

"Sometimes I feel like I must have done something bad to deserve this."

Are you asking yourself, "Why me?" Getting used to living with diabetes can be a challenge, and that's true whether you've just been diagnosed or you've lived with diabetes for a while.

About This Chapter: Information in this chapter is from "Diabetes: Dealing With Feelings." This information was provided by TeensHealth, one of the largest resources online for medically reviewed health information written for parents, kids, and teens. For more articles like this one, visit www.TeensHealth.org, or www.KidsHealth.org. © 2005 The Nemours Center for Children's Health Media, a division of The Nemours Foundation.

If You've Just Found Out You Have Diabetes

When people are first diagnosed with diabetes, they might be nervous about getting shots or medical tests and scared about how diabetes will affect their future health.

In the beginning, almost everyone thinks that they will never be able to do the blood sugar testing or insulin injections they need to stay healthy. But after working with doctors and learning more about diabetes, these things start feeling like less of a big deal. Over time, shots and checks can become like brushing teeth or taking a shower—just another daily routine you do to stay healthy. Eventually, some people even start to feel pretty good about the fact that they are able to do all the things they need to do to manage their diabetes on their own.

It's perfectly normal for people with diabetes to feel sad, angry, confused, upset, alone, embarrassed, and even jealous. After all, these are natural emotions that everyone feels from time to time. But how can you cope?

♣ It's A Fact!!

How well you cope with diabetes depends on how well you:

- Understand diabetes and how it affects your body.
- Understand how to control your blood glucose levels.
- Communicate with your health care provider.
- Understand the diabetes care plan developed with your health care provider.
- Understand the emotional ups and downs that come with having diabetes.
- Cope with stressful life events.
- Use family and social support systems.

Source: "Coping with Diabetes" by Raylene McCalman, MS, RD, LD, CDE, Extension Diabetes Coordinator, and Martha Archuleta, PhD, RD, Extension Food and Nutrition Specialist. © 2003 College of Agriculture and Home Economics Cooperative Extension Service, New Mexico State University.

Dealing With Your Feelings

Here are a few things you can do to cope with the emotional side of diabetes:

Open up to people you trust. If you feel sad, mad, embarrassed, or worried, talk about it with a close friend, parent, or doctor. It might be hard at first to open up, and you may have trouble finding the words to talk about it. Try to name your feelings and say what's got you feeling that way. Many times, just telling someone who will listen and understand your feelings can lighten a difficult emotion and help it to pass. Make it a regular habit to talk about what you're going through with someone close to you. As time goes on, be sure to notice and talk about the positive feelings, too. With time, you may notice that you're feeling more calm and confident, or that you're proud of what you're learning to do.

Get more support if you need it. If you're having a really tough time, or if you think you may be depressed, let an adult know. (Some signs that it might be depression are you're sleeping or eating all the time or not at all, or you feel sad or angry for long periods.) Sometimes people need the added support and care of a counselor or a mental health professional. Your doctor, parent, or another trusted adult can put you in touch with a counselor or other mental health professional who works with teens that have diabetes. Get all the support you need and deserve.

Learn how to take care of yourself. When you take good care of yourself and manage your diabetes, you will probably get sick less often, need fewer extra shots or tests, and be able to do the same activities as everyone else. When you can participate and feel well enough to get exercise (which is a great mood booster), you'll feel better, too.

If you're ready to take charge of tracking your blood sugar levels, adjusting and taking your insulin injections, and taking responsibility for preparing your meals and snacks, talk to your parents and doctor about how you can start making these changes. Again, taking charge of these practical tasks can give you more of a sense of control and power over diabetes. You might begin to feel proud—even amazed—that you're doing things you didn't think you'd be able to do.

Tell your teachers about your diabetes. Telling your teachers at school that you have diabetes can make things a little easier for you—for example, you might tell your teacher that you need to check your insulin or have a snack at a certain time each day. That way you can just leave class without drawing extra attention to yourself. If your teacher knows you have diabetes, he or she can also be on the lookout for symptoms of diabetes problems and can call for medical help if you need it.

If you're not sure how to bring it up on your own, or don't know what to say, ask your doctor to give you a note that covers the basics for your teacher. That can get the conversation between you and your teacher started.

Get organized. There can be a lot to keep track of if you have diabetes. How much insulin did you take this morning? What did you eat at school? Did you pack your medicines? Getting organized can help you feel less worried about how diabetes will affect your health. Every night before going to school or work, check to make sure you have the snacks and medicines you'll need for the next day. You'll begin to feel prepared and in charge.

Focus on your strengths. It's easy to get lost in all the negative ways diabetes affects your world. If you feel like diabetes is taking over your life, it can help to write down your strengths—and the stuff you love. Who are you? Are you a reader, a hockey player, a music lover, a math whiz, a spelling champ? Are you a son or daughter, a sister or brother, a grandchild, student, friend, baby sitter? Are you a future astronomer, teacher, doctor, or poet? Diabetes is really only a small part of who you are. Keep track of your dreams and hopes, and find time for the people and things you enjoy.

Stick to the plan. Lots of people who have diabetes get sick of dealing with it once in a while. And sometimes people who have learned to manage their illness feel so healthy and strong that they wonder whether they need to keep following their diabetes management plan. For example, you may wonder whether you can skip a meal when you're at the mall or check your blood sugar after the game instead of before. But skipping medicines, veering off the meal plan, or not checking your blood sugar can have disastrous results if you have diabetes. If you feel like throwing in the towel, talk to your doctor. He or she can help you find solutions that fit your life and help you stay healthy, too.

Take your time. Your feelings about diabetes will change over time—today you might feel worried about the future and different from your friends, but next year you might wonder why you were so upset. As you learn to manage diabetes on your own and take a more active role in your health, you may find it's a little easier dealing with the ups and downs of diabetes.

Your Family's Feelings

Just as you can get emotional about your diabetes, so can parents and other family members. Seeing a parent get upset can be hard. It can help to remind yourself that the diabetes is not your fault, nor is it your parents' fault. Just as you feel upset from time to time, it's natural for your parents to feel that way, too.

When a parent or other family member is worried, it may show up in strange ways. For example, a parent may get angry with a doctor. Or your mom or dad may constantly ask how you feel, whether you're eating right, and whether you've taken your medication. Sure, you understand that they are doing this because they love you. But it can help to explain how this makes you feel. Find a good time to talk about it calmly and openly. Sometimes family counseling or joining a family support group can help families work through the emotional ups and downs of dealing with diabetes.

Other family members like grandparents, aunts, and uncles may also want to know if you're feeling OK—and all this attention can feel like prying or nosiness, especially when you just want to be treated like everyone else. If you're close to the person, you may be able to talk to him or her about how you feel. If not, you may just have to let it go and realize that your relative is trying to show concern; even if it's done clumsily, it's an expression of caring.

You may envy a brother or sister who doesn't have diabetes, but your sibling may feel envious of you because of the extra attention you're getting. Again, it can help to talk about this openly—and recognize that your sibling's feelings may show up in strange ways, such as anger at you.

Your Friends

It's up to you whether you tell friends or classmates about your diabetes. For some people, opening up can help them feel less embarrassed. They don't have to worry what friends think when they see them doing things to take care of the diabetes—like checking blood sugar levels or wearing an insulin pump.

✔ Quick Tip

Meet The Challenge

Once you learn you have diabetes, many things in your life may change. Financial and emotional costs of diabetes self-care, medical treatment, physical disabilities, changes in lifestyle, or hospitalizations can be overwhelming at times. Being prepared for these changes can help you better meet the challenges of having diabetes. Learn all that you can about controlling diabetes, participate in your health care, keep a positive attitude, and you will meet the challenge.

Learn All You Can

Take advantage of chances to learn all you can about diabetes, how it affects your body, and what you need to do each day to control your blood glucose levels. Knowledge is power! Changes in your lifestyle—eating habits, exercise, blood glucose monitoring, medications, and more—need not be difficult or drastic. Contact hospitals and clinics in your area for information about group diabetes classes, workshops, or health fairs.

Be A Part Of The Team

You are not alone. Talk to your health care provider, dietitian, diabetes educator, and pharmacist whenever you have questions or concerns about diabetes, your medications, or your treatment plan. This team of health professionals is dedicated to helping you manage your diabetes. Be honest, ask questions, and participate in planning a diabetes treatment and self-care plan. Talking to your providers openly and taking an active role in making decisions about your health will help you be successful in managing your diabetes.

Build Coping Skills

Life can be challenging enough without the burden of a chronic disease like diabetes. How you handle the emotional ups and downs of living with

---

If you choose to tell your friends, be prepared for them to ask questions about what having diabetes means and how it makes you feel. Some of their questions may seem silly or funny to you. But ultimately, friends who know about your health problem can be a source of support as you deal with your feelings about diabetes. Having friends who are willing to listen when you're

diabetes and how you cope with stressful life events will be very personal. Learn strategies and skills to cope with daily challenges. Some people use prayer, exercise, meditation, or other forms of stress management. Take control of your daily life. Much of the stress in our lives comes from feeling overwhelmed by too many demands. Look for ways to reduce the demands on your time and make sure to take time each day for yourself. For help with learning how to deal with stress and diabetes, ask your health care provider about finding a mental health specialist who has experience working with people who have diabetes.

Family Support

People who have a strong support system in place tend to be healthier and recover quicker from illnesses. Without help and understanding from family and friends, you may feel alone and isolated when dealing with the daily demands of having diabetes. Keep family members involved in your diabetes management. Remember that many things you need to do to stay healthy are the same things your family should be doing now to prevent diabetes in the future. Lifestyle changes are easier when the entire family joins in. Diabetes support groups and group classes provide a chance to discuss problems with other people who have diabetes. Since diabetes affects the whole family, invite them to join you at classes and meetings. Health care providers or diabetes educators are available to answer specific questions you or your family may have.

Source: "Coping with Diabetes" by Raylene McCalman, MS, RD, LD, CDE, Extension Diabetes Coordinator, and Martha Archuleta, PhD, RD, Extension Food and Nutrition Specialist. © 2003 College of Agriculture and Home Economics Cooperative Extension Service, New Mexico State University.

depressed, angry, and frustrated—even if they don't have diabetes them-selves—can definitely help you feel better.

It's wise to be aware of how friends and family feel, but your first priority is dealing with your own emotions. The teen years can be an emotionally tough time to start with—hormones can put anyone's emotions on a roller coaster ride without adding a health condition to the mix.

It's only human to let off some steam if you're going through a difficult adjustment—like dealing with diabetes—and the strong feelings that go with it. But if you find your emotions are getting the best of you, if you're feeling really down or really angry, or if you're having a tough time managing your health routines, let your doctor know. Together, you can work out a plan for getting your situation under control.

It can take a long time to deal with having diabetes, and there's no set adjustment period—some people accept it and adapt quickly whereas others need more time. One thing's for sure, though: Even people who have lived with the condition for a while may still experience strong emotions, such as fear or sadness, from time to time or when faced with new situations. It's normal to feel overwhelmed occasionally.

Positive emotions can be part of the adjustment process, too. Don't be surprised if, as you adapt to your diabetes, you find yourself feeling proud, confident, determined, hopeful, interested, relieved, relaxed, loved, supported, strong—and yes, even happy. In time, you can become an expert at recogniz-ing and dealing with your emotions, and doing your part to care for your health. In fact, having diabetes might even teach you ways to cope with and adjust to life's ups and downs in a way that many teens can't.

Chapter 53

Depression And Diabetes

Introduction

Depression can strike anyone, but people with diabetes, a serious disorder that afflicts an estimated 16 million Americans, may be at greater risk. In addition, individuals with depression may be at greater risk for developing diabetes. Treatment for depression helps people manage symptoms of both diseases, thus improving the quality of their lives.

Several studies suggest that diabetes doubles the risk of depression compared to those without the disorder. The chances of becoming depressed increase as diabetes complications worsen. Research shows that depression leads to poorer physical and mental functioning, so a person is less likely to follow a required diet or medication plan. Treating depression with psychotherapy, medication, or a combination of these treatments can improve a patient's well being and ability to manage diabetes.

Causes underlying the association between depression and diabetes are unclear. Depression may develop because of stress but also may result from the metabolic effects of diabetes on the brain. Studies suggest that people with diabetes who have a history of depression are more likely to develop

About This Chapter: Information in this chapter is excerpted from "Depression And Diabetes," a publication of the National Institute of Mental Health (NIMH), National Institutes of Health (NIH), NIH Publication No. 02-5003, May 2002.

diabetic complications than those without depression. People who suffer from both diabetes and depression tend to have higher health care costs in primary care.

Despite the enormous advances in brain research in the past 20 years, depression often goes undiagnosed and untreated. People with diabetes, their families and friends, and even their physicians may not distinguish the symptoms of depression. However, skilled health professionals will recognize these symptoms and inquire about their duration and severity, diagnose the disorder, and suggest appropriate treatment.

Depression Facts

Depression is a serious medical condition that affects thoughts, feelings, and the ability to function in everyday life. Depression can occur at any age. National Institute of Mental Health–sponsored studies estimate that 6 percent of 9- to 17-year-olds in the U.S. and almost 10 percent of American adults, or about 19 million people age 18 and older, experience some form of depression every year. Although available therapies alleviate symptoms in over 80 percent of those treated, less than half of people with depression get the help they need.

Depression results from abnormal functioning of the brain. The causes of depression are currently a matter of intense research. An interaction between genetic predisposition and life history appears to determine a person's level of risk. Stress, difficult life events, side effects of medications, or other environmental factors may then trigger episodes of depression. Whatever its origins, depression can limit the energy needed to keep focused on treatment for other disorders, such as diabetes.

Get Treatment For Depression

While there are many different treatments for depression, they must be carefully chosen by a trained professional based on the circumstances of the person and family. Prescription antidepressant medications are generally well tolerated and safe for people with diabetes. Specific types of psychotherapy, or "talk" therapy, also can relieve depression. However, recovery from depression takes time. Antidepressant medications can take several weeks to

♣ It's A Fact!!
Symptoms Of Depression

- Persistent sad, anxious, or "empty" mood

- Feelings of hopelessness, pessimism

- Feelings of guilt, worthlessness, helplessness

- Loss of interest or pleasure in hobbies and activities that were once enjoyed, including sex

- Decreased energy, fatigue, being "slowed down"

- Difficulty concentrating, remembering, making decisions

- Insomnia, early-morning awakening, or oversleeping

- Appetite and/or weight changes

- Thoughts of death or suicide, or suicide attempts

- Restlessness, irritability

If five or more of these symptoms are present every day for at least two weeks and interfere with routine daily activities such as work, self-care, or social life, seek an evaluation for depression.

work and may need to be combined with ongoing psychotherapy. Not everyone responds to treatment in the same way. Prescriptions and dosing may need to be adjusted.

In people who have diabetes and depression, scientists report that psychotherapy and antidepressant medications have positive effects on both mood and glycemic control. Additional trials will help us better understand the links between depression and diabetes and the behavioral and physiologic mechanisms by which improvement in depression fosters better adherence to diabetes treatment and healthier lives.

A mental health professional—for example, a psychiatrist, psychologist, or clinical social worker—who is in close communication with the physician providing the diabetes care should manage treatment for depression in the context of diabetes. This is especially important when antidepressant medication is needed or prescribed, so that potentially harmful drug interaction can be avoided. In some cases, a mental health professional that specializes in treating individuals with depression and co-occurring physical illnesses such as diabetes may be available. People with diabetes who develop depression, as well as people in treatment for depression who subsequently develop diabetes, should make sure to tell any physician they visit about the full range of medications they are taking.

Use of herbal supplements of any kind should be discussed with a physician before they are tried. Recently, scientists have discovered that St. John's wort, an herbal remedy sold over-the-counter and promoted as a treatment for mild depression can have harmful interactions with some other medications.

Other mental disorders, such as bipolar disorder (manic-depressive illness) and anxiety disorders, may occur in people with diabetes, and they too can be effectively treated.

☞ Remember!!

Remember, depression is a treatable disorder of the brain. Depression can be treated in addition to whatever other illnesses a person might have, including diabetes. If you think you may be depressed or know someone who is, don't lose hope. Seek help for depression.

Chapter 54

Diabetes Burnout And Getting Back On Track

Diabetes burnout is a result of the never-ending, often overwhelming, constantly demanding and frustrating burden of diabetes self-care. People with diabetes burnout know that reasonable care is important for their health, but they just don't have the motivation to keep it up. It is one of the most common emotional challenges for people with diabetes, and most people with diabetes have periods of time where they feel burnout. Diabetes burnout is not necessarily the same as feeling depressed or in denial. It has more to do with feeling unmotivated, unable or unwilling to change, or just plain tired of the endless attention and effort required by diabetes or frustrated with the inevitable blood sugar fluctuations despite painstaking vigilance.

How to get back on track. Ask yourself what you need to do to get back on track. What barriers do you have to overcome? Where could you start? Define one thing you could do to start to improve your situation. Start with one of your easier challenges so that you have a greater chance of success.

Second, are there other people who could help you? Support at home, at work, and at play from family and friends will increase your chances of success.

About This Chapter: Information in this chapter is from "I Feel Burnt Out by Diabetes Care. Any Suggestions About How to Get Back on Track?" Copyright © 2005 by Joslin Diabetes Center. All rights reserved. Reprinted with permission from The Joslin Diabetes Center website, http://www.joslin.org.

Decide what kind of support you need and then tell the people who are involved with your care what you need. Don't forget your health care team. They are your partners in setting goals, overcoming barriers, and solving problems. Go see them more often, and arrange for more contact between visits, for example, through telephone calls or faxing blood glucose records.

Third, understand and tolerate that strong negative feelings about diabetes are normal and that these feelings are nothing to be ashamed of or guilty about. Many people speak of "accepting" diabetes—this does not mean liking diabetes, it means tolerating the hatred of diabetes enough to still take care of yourself. Talking with family, friends, health professionals or others with diabetes who understand these feelings can be helpful in learning how to cope with them in more constructive ways.

Fourth, keep your eye on the rewards of good care and what worked well, not the failures and the consequences. Fears about complications from diabetes may motivate you for a short period of time, but in the long run most people either rationalize consequences away or become paralyzed by fear. Rather, focus on the rewards of better care whatever they may be (quicker responses on the basketball court, fewer arguments at home, more productivity at work, improved concentration, for example) and remember what has worked well before and try it again.

Finally, engage in problem solving. First, try to concretely and specifically define the problem. Second, become aware of when, how, and where the problem occurs. Third, once the problem is defined then consider potential solutions. Consider changing your behavior or the environment to make it easier to deal with the problem. For example, if you are having trouble finding time to exercise, consider buying a treadmill for home rather than expecting you will find time to go to the gym. Keep in mind what you can learn from previous successes with a similar problem. Fourth, make life easier for yourself by avoiding the problem, if possible. This assumption goes directly against the great American myth

☞ Remember!!
Remember that motivation is fueled by success, but success depends upon having realistic, practical and achievable goals.

that "willpower" is the answer to life troubles and, in fact, assumes that self-discipline fails for almost everyone when exposed to enough temptation, lack of support or stress. For example, if you love to eat you should not find yourself in front of the all-you-can-eat buffet and naively expect that self-discipline will help control your overeating.

Chapter 55

Diabetes And Relationships

Studies indicate that one of the best predictors of how well people take care of their diabetes is the amount of support they get from their family and friends. However, not all support is helpful. For example, one person might appreciate his family watching everything he eats while that type of scrutiny might drive another person to the do the exact opposite.

How do you get the kind of support you need? First, you have to decide what, when, and how you want support. Then you need to tell the people who are involved with your care what you need. Usually, family members and friends are willing to help. If they have embarrassed or irritated you in the past, it might be that they don't understand diabetes, or they are not sure how to help. They simply did what they thought was helpful.

Therefore, you need to:

- Educate your family and friends about your diabetes.

- Define how you want family and friends to help.

- Ask them directly for help and teach them how to give it.

Second, family members and friends need to understand diabetes, listen to what you think and feel, and support or join you in making some healthy changes. For example, if you are trying to lose weight, it simply will be easier if your family also eats the same low-fat foods. Your family and friends may also have concerns and worries (for example, guilt, fear, anger, etc.) about your diabetes that need to be talked about so that realistic expectations can be set, misconceptions corrected, and feelings understood.

Perhaps the two most important guidelines for family members are to have realistic expectations about blood glucose levels and to avoid blame. Family members need your help and the help of your health care team in

---

✔ **Quick Tip**

When should I tell my date about diabetes?

You need to tell people that you have diabetes when you feel the time is right. If you treat your diabetes as a natural, everyday part of your life, your date will feel more comfortable asking and learning about it.

What should I share about low blood sugars?

It is important for your date to understand your reactions to low blood sugars. Tell your date what to do if you cannot treat yourself. Explain that these changes in behavior are not to be taken personally.

What should I tell the person I am dating about diabetes care?

Explain the connection between food, insulin, and blood sugar. Dispel the myth about what you can and cannot eat. If consuming alcohol, discuss how it may affect you. Discuss social situations that may arise, the importance of being prepared for the unexpected, and consequences if you are not. Situations that may arise include the following:

- Delayed dinners

- Effects of exercise

- Unplanned overnights

order to understand that you cannot always control blood glucose levels even if you follow your diabetes care plan. Blaming the person with diabetes for high or low blood glucose levels never helps and frequently causes hurt feelings, arguments or serious conflict. The key to genuine support is to avoid blame and focus on problem solving.

With that said, there are times when there may be no clue as to what has caused a problem with diabetes management or how to correct it. At moments like these, what may be needed is a hug, a sympathetic word or a dozen roses. Family and friends need to understand that this kind of support can be very helpful during frustrating times.

When should I include my significant other in the awareness of ongoing diabetes care responsibilities?

As your relationship becomes more serious, it is probably time for your significant other to understand the day-to-day things that you have to do to take care of yourself, such as:

- Blood sugar testing.
- Injections.
- Carrying supplies and food.
- Doctor appointments.
- Prescription refills.
- Sick day management.

Think about suggesting a meeting between the person you are dating and your parents, who have knowledge about your diabetes. Do not expect the significant other to learn everything in one day. It takes communication to become knowledgeable and supportive.

Source: "Dating? Engaged? Married?" © 2005 Children's Diabetes Foundation. All rights reserved. Reprinted with permission.

Chapter 56

Keeping Your Self-Esteem

Your Emotions

Being a teen is a lot like riding a roller coaster. It can be both lots of fun and very hard at the same time. As a teen, it is normal for you to:

- feel confused.

- have mood swings.

- worry that others won't accept you.

But just because being a teen is normal does not mean it is easy. It can be even harder when you are dealing with an illness or disability. There is a lot to learn when you have a health issue, but there are steps you can take to cope.

Feeling Good About Yourself

Being a teen brings all sorts of new thoughts and feelings about different parts of your life, such as how you feel about:

- your friends and other kids your age.

- how you are doing in school and in other activities.

About This Chapter: Excerpted from "Illness and Disability—Your Emotions," 4 Girls Health, U.S. Department of Health and Human Services, Office on Women's Health, May 2005.

- your parents.

- the way you look.

While having these new feelings, many changes are also taking place in your body. It is normal to feel self-conscious or shy about the changes in your body and emotions. Even though it might seem tough sometimes, remember that you are absolutely great!

Having a healthy or high self-esteem can help you to think positively, deal better with stress, and boost your drive to work hard. Having low self-esteem can cause you to feel uneasy and get in the way of doing things you might enjoy. For some, low self-esteem can lead to serious problems such as depression, drug and alcohol use, and eating disorders.

Find Out If You Have A Healthy Self-Esteem

If you have high or healthy self-esteem, you might think or say:

- I feel good about who I am.

- I am proud of what I can do, but I do not show off.

- I know there are some things that I am good at and some things I need to improve.

- I am responsible for the things I do and say, both good and bad.

- It is okay if I win or lose.

- Before I do something, I think "I can" and not, "I can't."

Does this sound like you? If only a few of the items in this list sound like you, that's okay—you're on the right track. Keep working at reminding yourself that you are a great person!

Find Out If You Have Low Or Poor Self-Esteem

If you have low or poor self-esteem, you might think or say:

- I can't do anything right.

- I am ugly or dumb.

- I do not have any friends.

- I do not like to try new things.

- It upsets me to make mistakes.

- I do not think I am as nice or as smart as the other kids in my class.

- I have a hard time making friends.

- I have a hard time making friends because I end up getting angry and fighting with people.

- It makes me uncomfortable when people say nice things about me.

- Sometimes I feel better if I say mean things to other people.

> ♣ **It's A Fact!!**
> **Self-Esteem**
>
> Self-esteem describes the value and respect you have for yourself. If you have a healthy self-esteem, you feel good about yourself as a person and are proud of what you can do. It is normal to have a hard time feeling good about yourself sometimes.

If many or all of these items sound like you, it will be helpful for you to work on having better self-esteem.

Steps To Better Self-Esteem

Try these steps to gain better self-esteem:

- Tell yourself that it is okay not to be the best at everything.

- Help out by doing chores around the house and volunteering in your community.

- Do things that you enjoy, or learn about new things you would like to try.

- Understand that there will be times when you will feel disappointed in yourself and other people. No one is perfect!

- If you are angry, try talking it over with an adult you trust (parents/ guardians or a school counselor).

- Think positively about yourself and the things you can do. Think: "I will try!"

- If you still find that you are not feeling good about yourself, talk to your parents, a school counselor, or your doctor because you may be at risk for depression. You can also ask the school nurse if your school offers counseling for help through tough times.

Chapter 57

Become A Diabetes Self-Advocate

As everyone with diabetes knows, much of the responsibility for diabetes care falls on the shoulders of the person who has it. You are in charge of monitoring your blood glucose every day, taking your insulin or oral drugs, choosing foods that fit your meal plan, and working exercise into your schedule. But even if you provide the bulk of your diabetes care, that doesn't mean you should have to manage your diabetes all alone. In fact, you really can't, which is why you should have a diabetes care team.

Your diabetes care team members are experts in different areas of diabetes management. Most teams have as a core group a doctor, a diabetes nurse educator, and a dietitian. Some other members you may have on your team include a mental health professional, ophthalmologist or optometrist, foot-care specialist, pharmacist, and exercise physiologist or physical therapist. Some people may also have a neurologist, kidney specialist, or any number of other medical specialists on the team. The list of team members can go on and on. The point, however, is that you are likely to have many people involved in your diabetes care. In general, that's a good thing. But it can be a challenge to get all your diabetes care team members to work together to achieve the best results.

About This Chapter: Information in this chapter is from "Several Habits of Highly Effective Self-Advocates." Reprinted with permission from Diabetes Self-Management. Copyright © 2001 R. A. Rapaport Publishing, Inc. For subscription information, call (800) 234-0923 or visit www.diabetesselfmanagement.com.

In an ideal world, all the members of your diabetes team would communicate with one another to coordinate your care and make sure that you get all the tests, checkups, education, and treatments that you need. If you needed to see a specialist not currently on your team, your primary care doctor would give you a referral, and your insurance company would cover the specialist's services.

In a more realistic world, your doctor may not practice in a diabetes care center that supports a team system. Your various health care providers may not communicate with each other. Your insurance company may not see the necessity of paying for visits to an exercise specialist or mental health professional. And you may find you have to remind your primary care provider to write you a referral to an eye doctor once a year or to examine your feet at every regular diabetes office visit.

The skills of self-advocacy seem to come naturally to some people. Many others, however, have to learn them. The good news is that the skills of self-advocacy can be learned, and it doesn't require a personality overhaul or assertiveness training courses.

One of the most important parts of self-advocacy is knowledge—of the latest guidelines for diabetes care, of what your health insurance plan covers, and of new diabetes treatments. Another part is becoming an expert on you and your diabetes by keeping records of your blood glucose levels and self-management routines. And another part is speaking up, including letting your health care providers know what's working and what's not.

Changing World, Changing Needs

Self-advocacy has always been important, but today it is perhaps more necessary than ever for two reasons: recent changes in the health care system and the ever-increasing number of options for the treatment of diabetes.

> ♣ **It's A Fact!!**
> In this more realistic world, you may have to be in charge of coordinating your care. That means you not only have to manage your diabetes on a day-to-day basis, but you also have to ensure that your medical and educational needs are being met. Some people call this being a self-advocate.

In the past decade or so, the health care system in the United States has changed phenomenally as insurance companies and the U.S. and state governments have tried to rein in health care spending. Fee-for-service plans are rapidly being replaced with health maintenance organizations, preferred provider organizations, and other managed care plans. In the old system, health care consumers often had minimal responsibility for the course of their treatment. In the new system, it helps a lot to know what resources are available to you and how to access them.

New treatment options for people with diabetes include new drugs, new insulins, and new methods of insulin delivery. Guidelines for diet and exercise have evolved, too, in recent years. These developments bode well for improved blood glucose control, but they can also mean that new information must be learned and new skills acquired. Making sure you get the information, education, and skills training you need to take advantage of new treatment options may require using many of the skills of self-advocacy.

Start With Knowledge

As a participant in your treatment plan, it's helpful to learn as much as possible about prudent diabetes care and your own treatment options.

The ADA recommends that all people with diabetes have their weight, blood pressure, and feet checked at each scheduled diabetes care visit. Are you getting these basic exams? An easy way to remind your health care provider to check your feet is to take off your shoes and socks as soon as you go into the exam room.

The ADA also recommends a glycosylated hemoglobin (HbA1c) test approximately every three months. The HbA1c test gives an indication of your average level of blood glucose control over the preceding two to three months. It is a useful tool for determining whether your diabetes care plan is doing the job or needs adjustments.

✔ Quick Tip

To get a general sense of what your medical care should include, take a look at the guidelines developed by the American Diabetes Association (ADA) to maintain optimal health and help prevent complications.

A lipid profile, including total cholesterol level, LDL cholesterol level, HDL cholesterol level, and triglycerides, is recommended annually to assess your risk for heart disease and need for treatment. Some other tests that are recommended on an annual basis are a dilated eye exam, dental exam, and a test for microalbuminuria, an early sign of kidney damage. The ADA also recommends getting a flu shot every year to prevent the flu and its complications.

The ADA guidelines are general guidelines and may be modified by your health care team. Specific recommendations for medicines, meal planning, exercise, and blood glucose monitoring should be tailored to you, as well.

Know Your Treatment Options

Becoming familiar with available medicines will help you and your doctor choose what is best for you. For people with Type 2 diabetes, there are now drugs that increase insulin secretion, including sulfonylureas (chlorpropamide, glimepiride, glipizide, glyburide, tolazamide, and tolbutamide) as well as nateglinide and repaglinide; drugs that decrease absorption of glucose in the digestive tract (acarbose and miglitol); a drug that decreases the release of glucose by the liver (metformin); and drugs that help reverse insulin resistance (pioglitazone and rosiglitazone). All of these may be prescribed alone or in combination with certain other drugs.

For people who require insulin, there are also choices, including long-acting insulin, intermediate-acting insulin, short-acting insulin, and rapid-acting insulin. There is also the choice between animal-derived insulin, genetically engineered human insulin, and insulin analogs, which are similar to but slightly different from human insulin.

Before you ask your doctor for the latest product, think about whether and why you need a change. Some questions to ask yourself include the following:

- Am I achieving target ranges for my blood sugar with my current drug or insulin regimen?

- Is my HbA1c test result below 7%, the goal set out by the ADA?

✔ Quick Tip

How do you know what's new on the market and what might work for you? Read books, journals, and newsletters. Visit reliable Web sites, and make a list of online resources that you visit regularly. Attend diabetes classes and seminars, watch for engagements with speakers you can learn from, join a support group, and develop the art of networking in the diabetes community.

- Am I able to take my pills or insulin at the times suggested?

- Have I experienced any side effects with my current regimen?

- Will the new pill or insulin I'm interested in taking be safe for me? (This may depend on whether you have other medical conditions such as kidney or liver disease.)

- Will a new pill or insulin have any particular benefit over what I'm using now?

Meal planning and exercise are equally important parts of managing diabetes, and there are many approaches to both. If you do not yet have an individualized meal plan or are having trouble with the one you have, request an appointment with a dietitian. Speak to your doctor about safe forms of exercise for you. Choose a program that you can commit to with consistency and that takes into consideration your lifestyle and personal likes and dislikes.

Blood glucose monitoring is recommended for everyone who has diabetes, but the frequency with which you monitor may depend on how you treat your diabetes and other factors. If you are newly diagnosed with diabetes, your blood sugar is unstable, or you use insulin, you will probably want to check more often. In general, you want to check often enough to get the information you need to make daily diabetes self-management decisions. Your health care team can help you choose a meter, determine how often to use it each day, and determine the best times of day to check your blood glucose.

Know Your Insurance Coverage

The documents provided by insurance companies will never be mistaken for great literature, but it's worth making the effort to slog through them anyway. Whether you have a choice of policy or not, it's important to know what's covered and what's not. For example, what is the prescription coverage? Are most of your prescription needs on the drug formulary, and if not, what are the costs of nonformulary items? Will you need a doctor's letter of necessity to help you obtain them? Are there limits on diabetes supplies? What is the copayment for doctor visits? Will you be able to see your doctor when you want to? What is the procedure for being referred to a specialist?

Some other questions to investigate include these: What are the limits on emergency room or hospital visits? What if you have a medical problem when you are away from home? What procedures require pre-authorization? What is the appeals process for denied claims? (All insurance companies have one.)

If you are confused by what you read, call the insurance company's customer service number with questions. You might also seek help from someone in your company's human resources department if you get your health insurance coverage through your job.

Once you have insurance coverage, keep in mind that your insurance company's policies are subject to change, so if you're scheduled for an expensive procedure, it doesn't hurt to check and double check what's covered. When Jessica had her first vitrectomy, she didn't need pre-authorization from the insurance company before the procedure. So when she was scheduled for a second vitrectomy, she didn't think she'd need pre-authorization for it, either. But she asked the office manager of her retinal specialist to call and confirm coverage anyway. As it turned out, a requirement for pre-authorization had been implemented the month before. If Jessica had not checked, she could have been responsible for a substantial bill.

If you receive a bill or a reimbursement check that doesn't seem right, call your insurance company immediately. Don't let it sit around and gather dust.

> ☞ **Remember!!**
>
> Your daily diabetes management routine—including taking medicines, planning meals, exercising, and checking blood glucose levels—can only be effective if you follow it consistently. Don't wait to become "motivated." Motivation comes from the self-confidence you gain and the payoff you reap when you initiate action. If something in your plan doesn't seem to be working, contact your health care provider to discuss possible alternatives.

And don't hesitate to use the appeals process for denied claims when you disagree with a decision. If you call the insurance company but seem to be getting nowhere, ask to speak to a supervisor. Document all calls with the date, time, person you spoke to, and the matter discussed.

Carlos learned all of these lessons and more when a human error put his insurance coverage in jeopardy. Carlos had a work-related disability and wanted to make sure his insurance continued until he got back to work. He talked to his employer, the disability caseworker, the workman's compensation case coordinator, and an insurance company representative to confirm continued coverage. Everything was set, or so he thought, until he started receiving medical bills. He repeated his calls, but no one could tell him what had happened, and no one had the authority to re-instate coverage.

Carlos kept calling until finally an insurance representative checked her computer records carefully. She saw that a wrong code had been entered but said the only person who could change it was the person who had typed it in, and she didn't know who that was. Carlos explained the gravity of his situation forcefully, but politely. She asked him to hold for a minute, then came back to report the code had been corrected, and coverage was intact. Sometimes, persistence is the key.

Become An Expert On You

A good self-advocate must also be a good historian and record keeper. You and your diabetes team cannot design a plan specifically for you if there is not enough information on which to base decisions.

An important but oft-neglected record is a personal list of medicines, doses, and times taken. Keep your list up to date, and keep it in a place such as your wallet, where it is readily available for appointments with members of your health care team. It is also wise to make a copy for a close friend or family member in the event of an emergency.

Your list of medicines will come in handy should you have to fill out a medical history questionnaire. There are some other details you'll want to have written down, too, such as the date of your most recent chest x-ray, the dates of any surgeries, highlights of your and your family's medical history, insurance information, and the names and addresses of members of your diabetes team and other health care providers. The more complicated your medical history, the more difficult it is to remember things.

Blood glucose self-monitoring records are essential to assess how your treatment plan is working. Log books, meter memory, and downloading programs are all designed to make this easier. Be sure to take your blood glucose monitoring records with you to all your appointments.

Speak Up

Being aware of treatment plan options and keeping records are of little help if you are unable to ask questions or share concerns. But speaking up can be intimidating for many people. If you feel that way, remember to give yourself credit for what you know: You are the expert of your own body. Remember, too, that you're paying for a service. If possible, find a doctor who doesn't make you feel rushed or uncomfortable. Speaking up may take practice, but with time, it will get less scary and feel more natural.

> **✔ Quick Tip**
>
> Wearing a medical ID is also a form of self-advocacy. In an emergency, you might be misdiagnosed or given inappropriate care if vital information about you is not available. A medical ID is an inexpensive investment when compared to the risk of receiving the wrong treatment.

To get the most out of a doctor visit or an appointment with another health care professional, it helps if you know what you want from it. Perhaps you're seeking relief from a particular symptom. Or maybe you have some questions about the drugs you're taking or about a new drug you've heard about. Formulate a list of priorities and questions ahead of time, and bring the list with you to your appointment. Bring a notebook, too, to jot down your doctor's answers or other information you want to retain. If you have a lot to discuss, you may be able to request a longer appointment. Most providers will appreciate your attitude of collaboration.

Have your personal documentation ready and in order for health care appointments. Bring your blood glucose monitoring records, insulin dosage records, food diary or carbohydrate intake log, exercise schedule, and any articles or clippings that have triggered questions. Collect what you need several hours before your appointment rather than as you are running out the door.

The information you provide needs to be accurate and truthful. If it is not, your care may suffer. George told his nurse practitioner that he had not eaten in the previous eight hours when she drew blood for a fasting blood sugar check. In fact, he had had a regular soft drink on his way to the clinic, and it showed in his blood glucose level. But because his nurse practitioner thought he was fasting (and George had brought no blood glucose monitoring records to refer to) she doubled his dose of medicine.

Immediately after his visit to the nurse practitioner, George saw the clinic dietitian and complained of symptoms of hypoglycemia in the mornings. When she asked how he had coped with skipping breakfast for his fasting blood sugar check, he remembered the soft drink on the way to the clinic and told her about it. If she had not called the nurse practitioner and canceled the new prescription, George could have developed dangerously low blood sugar.

A Right And A Responsibility

Did you know you already have a Patient's Bill of Rights? It was developed in 1973 and revised in 1992 by the American Hospital Association, a national organization that represents hospitals, health care networks, and their patients. Among other things, the Patient's Bill of Rights lists a person's right to considerate and respectful care, adequate information to make decisions about treatment, privacy, access to medical records, and confidentiality. You will find the Bill of Rights posted in hospital and clinic settings. In addition, many states require that hospitals give people a copy of these rights when they are admitted to the hospital.

As a self-advocate, you also have the right—and the responsibility—to investigate different health plans, doctors, and clinics before choosing one. Need surgery? Compare surgeons, talk to people who have undergone the same surgery, and get a second opinion if you are unsure of its necessity.

Learn what you can about all aspects of your health care and diabetes care. Each day brings a new development in diabetes care, and remaining up to date means actively pursuing your diabetes education.

As you learn more about diabetes and its care, set personal goals, and ask your health care team to help you make a plan for meeting them. If you have abandoned any aspects of your self-management plan over the years, your goals might start with the commitment to get back to the basics of diabetes self-care. You may resolve to start checking your blood sugar regularly or to look into diabetes education classes in your area.

Self-advocacy means using all the resources available to see that your health needs are met. It is a skill for survival. More important, it is one of the keys to quality of life. As you learn to be your own self-advocate, share what you've learned with others. See to it that not everybody has to learn the hard way.

Part Six

If You Need More Information

Chapter 58

Additional Reading About Diabetes

Books

American Diabetes Association Complete Guide to Diabetes, 4th Edition
American Diabetes Association, Alexandria, VA; July 2005
ISBN: 1580402372

Conquering Diabetes
Anne L. Peters, Mark Harmel (Photographer)
Penguin Group, New York, NY; April 2005
ISBN: 1594630038

Diabetes
Carol McCormick Semple, Jerrold S. Olshan
Enslow Publishers, Inc., Berkeley Heights, NJ; October 2000
ISBN: 0766016609

Diabetes: The Ultimate Teen Guide
Katherine J. Moran, Lisa P. Merriman (Illustrator)
Rowman & Littlefield Publishers, Inc., Lanham, MD; January 2004
ISBN: 0810848066

Diabetes Sourcebook, 3rd Edition
Dawn D. Matthews
Omnigraphics, Inc., Detroit, MI; March 2003
ISBN: 0780806298

The Diabetic Athlete: Prescription for Exercise
Sheri Colberg
Human Kinetics Publishers, Champaign, IL; September 2000
ISBN: 0736032711

A Field Guide to Type 1 Diabetes, 2nd Edition
American Diabetes Association, Alexandria, VA; October 2002
ISBN: 1580401708

487 Really Cool Tips for Kids with Diabetes
Bo Nasmyth Loy, Spike Nasmyth Loy
American Diabetes Association, Alexandria, VA; December 2003
ISBN: 1580401910

Getting a Grip on Diabetes: Quick Tips for Kids
Spike Nasmyth Loy, Bo Nasmyth Loy
American Diabetes Association, Alexandria, VA; November 2000
ISBN: 1580400531

Guide to Healthy Restaurant Eating, 2nd Edition
Hope S. Warshaw
American Diabetes Association, Alexandria, VA; April 2002
ISBN: 158040152X

In Control: A Guide for Teens with Diabetes for Eli Lilly
Jean Betschart-Roemer, Susan Thom
Wiley, John & Sons, Inc., Hoboken, NJ; October 2001
ISBN: 0471212601

Insulin
Janice Yuwiler
Thomson Gale, Farmington Hills, MI; June 2005
ISBN: 1560069309

Mastering Your Diabetes: A Simple Plan for Taking Control of Your Health...and Your Life
American Diabetes Association, Alexandria, VA; April 2003
ISBN: 1580401570

1001 Tips for Living Well with Diabetes
American Diabetes Association, Alexandria, VA; August 2004
ISBN: 1580402186

Pumping Insulin: Everything You Need for Success with an Insulin Pump, 3rd Edition
John T. Walsh, Ruth Roberts
Torrey Pines Press, San Diego, CA; June 2000
ISBN: 1884804845

Type 1 Diabetes: A Guide for Children, Adolescents, Young Adults and Their Caregivers
Ragnar Hanas
Avalon Publishing Group, Emeryville, CA; January 2005
ISBN: 1569243964

Type 2 Diabetes in Teens: Secrets for Success
Jean Betschart-Roemer
Wiley, John & Sons, Inc., Hoboken, NJ; June 2002
ISBN: 0471150568

Articles

"A Better Way To Manage Childhood Diabetes," by Steven Gutierrez, in *Parenting*, November 1, 2004, Page 40.

"At-Risk Kids Focus Of Diabetes Study," by Warren King, in *The Seattle Times*, November 12, 2004.

"Diabesity: The New Childhood Epidemic," by Julie A. Evans, in *Prevention*, December 2003, Page 106.

"Diabetes: Are You At Risk?" by Sara Francis Fujimura, in *Science World*, November 17, 2003, Page 8.

"Diabetes Cure Found?" by Denise Faustman, in *Current Science*, January 21, 2005, Page 15.

"Diabetes' Littlest Victims: Youth Advocate Recounts His Life with the Disease and His Hope for the Future," by Gilles Attipoe, in *Ebony*, March 2005, Page 134.

"Heart Threat," in *Prevention*, June 2003, Page 160.

"Impaired Glucose Tolerance in Obese Children and Adolescents," in *Nutrition Research Newsletter*, April 2002, Page 6.

"In Defiance of Odds, 3 Sisters Have Type 1 Diabetes," by Susanne Quick, in *Milwaukee Journal Sentinel*, October 7, 2005.

"Initiative Launched to Provide Personal Health Records to Kids with Diabetes," in *Life Science Weekly*, November 16, 2004, Page 417.

"Insulin Resistance in Teens Raises High Blood Pressure Risk As Adults," in *Life Science Weekly*, November 2, 2004, Page 696.

"Kids with Diabetes and Other Endocrine Disorders Face More Bullying Than Others," in *Life Science Weekly*, December 28, 2004, Page 110.

"New Hope for Type 1 Diabetes," in *Prevention*, March 2005, Page 58.

"Prevalence of the Metabolic Syndrome Among U.S. Adolescents Rising," in *Life Science Weekly*, October 26 2004, Page 345.

"Safe at School Campaign Launched for Kids with Diabetes," in *Life Science Weekly*, November 2, 2004, Page 381.

"Study Shows Ease of Introducing Technology to Kids with Diabetes," in *Life Science Weekly*, November 16, 2004, Page 359.

"Tight Control Okay for Kids," by Paula Rasich, in *Prevention*, September 2003, Page 164.

"What About Diabetics in Schools? Is Student Care Adequate?" in *Ebony*, March 2005, Page 140.

Web-Based Documents

Alcohol, Tobacco, & Drugs
American Diabetes Association
Web page for this document: http://www.diabetes.org/for-parents-and-kids/for-teens/alcohol-tobacco-drugs.jsp

Dating and Diabetes
American Diabetes Association
Web page for this document: http://www.diabetes.org/for-parents-and-kids/for-teens/dating.jsp

Driving
American Diabetes Association
Web page for this document: http://www.diabetes.org/for-parents-and-kids/for-teens/driving.jsp

A Guide to Eating Out
Canadian Diabetes Association
Web page for this document: http://www.diabetes.ca/Section_About/eatingout.asp

Healthcare Team
Bayer HealthCare
Web page for this document: http://www.bayercarediabetes.com/diabcare/controlling/healthcareTeam/index.asp

Keeping Track of Your Blood Sugar
Nemours Foundation
Web page for this document: http://www.kidshealth.org/teen/diabetes_basics/what/track_blood_sugar.html

Sick Days
Royal Children's Hospital
Web page for this document: http://www.rch.org.au/diabetesmanual/manual.cfm?doc_id=2742

Sports, Exercise, and Diabetes
Nemours Foundation
Web page for this document: http://www.kidshealth.org/teen/
managing_diabetes/living/sports_diabetes.html

Type 1 Diabetes
American Diabetes Association
Web page for this document: http://www.diabetes.org/type-1-diabetes.jsp

Chapter 59

Directory Of Diabetes Resources

Federal Agencies

Centers for Disease Control and Prevention (CDC)
Division of Diabetes Translation
P.O. Box 8728
Silver Spring, MD 20910
Toll Free: 877-CDC-DIAB
Phone: 770-488-5000; Fax: 770-488-5966
Website: http://www.cdc.gov/diabetes
E-mail: diabetes@cdc.gov

Indian Health Service (IHS)
Indian Health Service National Diabetes Program
5300 Homestead Road, NE
Albuquerque, NM 87110
Phone: 505-248-4182; Fax: 505-248-4188
Website: http://www.ihs.gov
E-mail: diabetesprogram@mail.ihs.gov

About This Chapter: This list of organizations to contact for more information about diabetes and related health concerns was compiled from many sources deemed reliable. All contact information was verified in September 2005.

National Diabetes Education Program
1 Diabetes Way
Bethesda, MD 20892-3600
Toll Free: 800-438-5383; Phone: 301-496-3583
Website: http://ndep.nih.gov
E-mail: ndep@info.nih.gov

National Diabetes Information Clearinghouse
1 Information Way
Bethesda, MD 20892-3560
Toll Free: 800-860-8747; Fax: 703-738-4929
Website: http://diabetes.niddk.nih.gov
E-mail: ndic@info.niddk.nih.gov

National Eye Institute (NEI)
National Eye Health Education Program
2020 Vision Place
Bethesda, MD 20892-3655
Phone: 301-496-5248; Fax: 301-402-1065
Website: http://www.nei.nih.gov
E-mail: 2020@nei.nih.gov

National Heart, Lung, and Blood Institute (NHLBI) Information Center
P.O. Box 30105
Bethesda, MD 20824-0105
Phone: 301-592-8573; Fax: 240-629-3246; TTY: 240-629-3255
Website: http://www.nhlbi.nih.gov
E-mail: NHLBIinfo@rover.nhlbi.nih.gov

National Institute of Diabetes and Digestive and Kidney Diseases (NIDDK)
National Institutes of Health
Building 31; Room 9A04 Center Drive; MSC 2560
Bethesda, MD 20892-2560
Website: http://www.niddk.nih.gov

National Kidney and Urologic Diseases Information Clearinghouse (NKUDIC)
3 Information Way
Bethesda, MD 20892-3580
Toll Free: 800-891-5390; Fax: 703-738-4929
Website: http://kidney.niddk.nih.gov
E-mail: nkudic@info.niddk.nih.gov

National Institute of Dental and Craniofacial Research
National Institutes of Health
Bethesda, MD 20892-2190
Phone: 301-402-7364
Website: http://www.nidcr.nih.gov
E-mail: nidcrinfo@mail.nih.gov

Office of Minority Health Resource Center (OMH-RC)
P.O. Box 37337
Washington, DC 20013-7337
Toll Free: 800-444-6472; Fax: 301-251-2160
Website: http://www.omhrc.gov
E-mail: info@omhrc.gov

Weight-control Information Network (WIN)
1 Win Way
Bethesda, MD 20892-3665
Toll Free: 877-946-4627; Phone: 202-828-1025; Fax: 202-828-1028
Website: http://www.win.niddk.nih.gov
E-mail: win@info.niddk.nih.gov

Private Organizations

American Association of Diabetes Educators
100 W. Monroe Street, Suite 400
Chicago, IL 60603
Toll Free: 800-338-3633; Phone: 703-620-3660; Fax: 312-424-2427
Website: http://www.diabeteseducator.org

American Diabetes Association
1701 North Beauregard Street
Alexandria, VA 22311
Toll Free: 800-342-2383
Website: http://www.diabetes.org
E-mail: AskADA@diabetes.org

American Dietetic Association
120 South Riverside Plaza, Suite 2000
Chicago, IL 60606-6995
Toll Free: 800-877-1600
Website: http://www.eatright.org

American Urological Association Foundation
1128 North Charles Street
Baltimore, MD 21201
Toll Free: 800-242-2383; Phone: 410-468-1800
Website: http://www.afud.org
E-mail: admin@afud.org

American Podiatric Medical Association (APMA)
9312 Old Georgetown Road
Bethesda, MD 20814-1698
Toll Free :800-FOOTCARE
Phone: 301-581-9200; Fax: 301-530-2752
Website: http://www.apma.org
E-mail: askapma@apma.org

Canadian Diabetes Association
National Life Building
1400-522 University Ave.
Toronto, ON M5G 2R5
Toll Free: 800-226-8464
Phone: 416-363-0177; Fax: 416-408-7117
Website: http://www.diabetes.ca
E-mail: info@diabetes.ca

Children's Diabetes Foundation of the North Bay

128 Saratoga Court
Petaluma, CA 94954
Phone: 707-782-0774; Fax: 707-766-9699
Website: http://www.cdfnb.org

Diabetes Action Research and Education Foundation

426 C Street, NE
Washington, DC 20002
Phone: 202-333-4520; Fax: 202-558-5240
Website: http://www.diabetesaction.org
E-mail: info@diabetesaction.org

Diabetes Exercise and Sports Association (DESA)

8001 Montcastle Dr.
Nashville, TN 37221
Toll Free: 800-898-4322; Fax: 615-673-2077
Website: http://www.diabetes-exercise.org
E-mail: desa@diabetes-exercise.org

Joslin Diabetes Center

One Joslin Place
Boston, MA 02215
Phone: 617-732-2400
Website: http://www.joslin.org

Juvenile Diabetes Research Foundation International

120 Wall Street
New York, NY 10005-4001
Toll Free: 800-533-CURE (2873); Fax: 212-785-9595
Website: http://www.jdrf.org
E-mail: info@jdrf.org

National Kidney Foundation, Inc. (NKF)
30 East 33rd Street
New York, NY 10016
Toll-Free: 800-622-9010
Phone: 212-889-2210; Fax: 212-689-9261
Website: http://www.kidney.org
E-mail: info@kidney.org

Pedorthic Footwear Association (PFA)
7150 Columbia Gateway Drive, Suite G
Columbia, MD 21046-1151
Toll Free: 800-673-8447
Phone: 410-381-7278; Fax: 410-381-1167
Website: http://www.pedorthics.org
E-mail: info@pedorthics.org

Index

Index

Page numbers that appear in *Italics* refer to illustrations. Page numbers that have a small 'n' after the page number refer to information shown as Notes at the beginning of each chapter. Page numbers that appear in **Bold** refer to information contained in boxes on that page (except Notes information at the beginning of each chapter).